W9-AQO-496

TAKING ON
HEART
DISEASE

LARRY KING

Peggy Fleming, Brian Littrell, Mike Ditka,
Walter Cronkite, Joyce Carol Oates, Eddie Griffin,
Mike Wallace, Kate Jackson, Ed Bradley, Tommy Lasorda,
Pat Buchanan, Victoria Gotti, Regis Philbin, and Others...

Reveal How They Triumphed Over the Nation's #1 Killer
And How You Can, Too

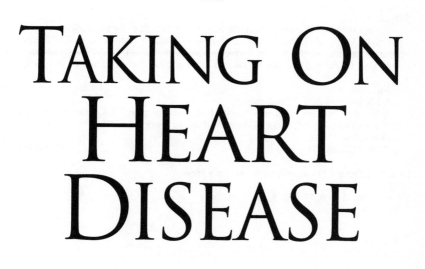

TAKING ON
HEART
DISEASE

RODALE

© 2004 by Spotlight Health

All rights reserved. No part of this publication may be reproduced or transmitted in any form or by any means, electronic or mechanical, including photocopying, recording, or any other information storage and retrieval system, without the written permission of the publisher.

Printed in the United States of America
Rodale Inc. makes every effort to use acid-free ∞, recycled paper ♻.

Photography credits appear on page 276.

Book design by Christina Gaugler

Library of Congress Cataloging-in-Publication Data

King, Larry.
    Taking on heart disease : Peggy Fleming, Brian Littrell, Mike Ditka, Walter Cronkite, Joyce Carol Oates, Eddie Griffin, Mike Wallace, Kate Jackson, Ed Bradley, Tommy Lasorda, Pat Buchanan, Victoria Gotti, Regis Philbin, and others . . . reveal how they triumphed over the nation's #1 killer and how you can, too / Larry King.
        p.   cm.
    Includes index.
    ISBN 1–57954–820–2 hardcover
    1. Heart—Diseases—Patients—United States—Biography. 2. Celebrities—United States—Biography. 3. Heart—Diseases—Popular works. I. Title.
RC666.7.K54   2004
362.196'612'0092273—dc22   2004000325

Distributed to the book trade by St. Martin's Press

2 4 6 8 10 9 7 5 3 1   hardcover

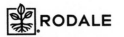

RODALE

WE INSPIRE AND ENABLE PEOPLE TO IMPROVE
THEIR LIVES AND THE WORLD AROUND THEM

FOR MORE OF OUR PRODUCTS
www.RODALESTORE.com
(800) 848-4735

To my brother, Marty Zeiger, who knows what it's like to go through bypass surgery and to be treated by the same doctors who helped me so much. He knows full well that all things are possible in this era of modern medicine.

Contents

PART III

This next segment of Larry's story includes
memories of his physical and spiritual recovery
after surgery.

P A R T I V

Surviving and Thriving 209
In this final segment, Larry explains what it means
to be a survivor of heart disease.

FOREWORD

Ten months after Larry King had what his friends now call "The Heart Attack," I performed quintuple bypass surgery on him to repair the plumbing in this vital organ. Since that day, he's been enjoying the most productive years of his life. In fact, just a few months ago, Larry celebrated his 70th birthday. He's convinced he wouldn't have lived to see any of this had he not made some changes to his lifestyle. He's right.

But when I first met him a few days before the surgery, Larry was like anyone else in this situation: nervous and scared about what was going to happen. I pulled up a chair. "My job is similar to finding a way out of a traffic jam on the Long Island Expressway," I told him. "Traffic can't move, so I'm going to make a detour around it. That's a bypass. And if you aren't nervous about what I'm going to do, you need a psychiatrist as well as a cardiac surgeon." I have always been aware there's not a single thing I can say that is going to take away the fear that patients feel, but I do tell them that when they walk out the door of this hospital in a few days, they'll be saying, "I got through this, and I'm doing okay." That's not a spiel. It's what I believe.

Since then, I've been on Larry's CNN program numerous times to talk about the body's remarkable pump. Heart disease kills almost half of the more than one million people who are diagnosed with it every year. And like any other disease, it doesn't care about your occupation, W2 form, age, or religion. Some of us are born with it; most of us develop it. But the primary reason the heart is taken for granted by all of us is a simple one: It works well. Out of sight, out of mind. That is, until something goes wrong.

Before Larry's surgery, the head of our hospital's neurology department stopped by his room to say hello and tell Larry how much he enjoyed his television show. He would later tell me in between department meetings that he had asked Larry why it's always the cardiologist who gets the praise when a brain surgeon could make one slip with a scalpel and the patient could lose his memory? Larry told him, "Well, nobody ever wrote a song called 'I Left My Brain in San Francisco.'" The neurosurgeon never brought up the issue again. But I did mention that conversation on the air with Larry when a caller asked what I thought was the most efficient and hard-working organ in the human body. I told him it's the heart, without question.

Yes, I have reason to be biased. I hold a human heart in my hands almost every day. And whenever I do, I marvel at how it is only about the size of two fists, yet it works every second of a person's life. It can react to illness or activity; it can withstand abuse from our lifestyle and genes; and, usually, it continues pumping almost 6 liters of blood every minute through miles and miles of vessels and arteries, without fail.

But it doesn't always do that. In the pages that follow, you will step into the lives of some of the busiest people on the planet—people who have had to come to a sudden and complete stop. Heart disease is never on The Schedule. And during that momentary pause, each person came to realize that what they do for a living isn't as important as what they can do to *keep* living. In some of the stories, a new lifestyle has been the result (and Larry's the poster boy for that). In others, a decision is made to just not get as wound up about things as before.

The onset of any disease requires us to react in four ways: to pay attention to the warning signs and symptoms; to get a diagnosis and understand the treatment options; to work through the recovery process; and to understand that the world will continue, and we must accept and make the lifestyle changes that are necessary to allow us to be a part of it. *Taking On Heart Disease* is divided into the same four steps, so you can better understand the journey. Facing disease can be humbling, because each person has to look at that proverbial Big Picture and decide how he or she fits, or *will* fit in the future. Yet the experience can also be enlightening: People can make changes in the way they've done things prior to surgery that allow them to remain productive. In fact, in many cases, they are *more productive* after surgery than before they were diagnosed. I see it every day.

Today, we are smarter about heart disease, both as doctors and as patients. Since the days not so long ago when Larry had The Heart Attack, treatments have improved for patients in both the emergency room and the operating room. And more exciting changes are on the way. I think in the years to come, we will be less likely to open a patient's chest to fix a heart in need of repair. Instead, it will be done through a catheter in an artery using robotics. In fact, that's happening right now.

Further, patients today are more educated about what has happened to them, how it happened, and maybe most important, how to keep it from happening again. I am convinced medicine is going to find the unknowns out there about why one person's heart falters while another person with a similar background has a heart that performs perfectly. It's going to be something we haven't thought about. My own theory is that perhaps the disease we see later in life may be the cumulative result of injuries or viruses that we faced when we were children. And if a person smokes or has high blood pressure or high cholesterol, that accelerates the changes. Perhaps the definitive answer will come to us through a long-term research study, or perhaps we'll stumble upon it accidentally. It may be staring us in the face right now and nobody is putting it together. After all, there are three arteries supplying the heart, but when I operate on someone, the arteries don't all look the same. For instance, someone will come in with one of those arteries 99 percent blocked. Yet the other two vessels are in perfect condition. And the parts before the blockage and after the blockage are so clean they look like they belong to a baby. But there's one blockage. Now why is it just in that one vessel? There is something else going on in the heart that we have yet to understand. But we will.

Don't wait for medicine to come up with the answer, however. Begin with your children. That's the take-home message for everyone. Even at age 10, children understand (I know this from first-hand experience with my own kids) what a lousy diet and lack of exercise can do to the body. If a child is aware of what happens, the adult who follows will be healthier. This should be a part of every elementary school science class. We'll never eliminate heart disease, but each one of us—as these stories prove—has a role in what happens to us as we get older.

You may be holding this book because you have just been told you have heart disease. Or, maybe, you are a family member or a friend of someone with heart disease. Maybe you are concerned about the risk factors (such as genetics, diet, and smoking, to name a few) that have been directly linked to heart damage. In the pages to come, Larry takes us through his experience with a disease that will never leave his body. He also brings you the stories of others whose names and work we know, people who faced the very real possibility that life could end sooner than they ever expected. These are stories from the front lines about the will to live. As you'll soon see, each of these people handled heart disease differently, but today, all are making plans for tomorrow.

O. Wayne Isom, M.D.
Chairman of Cardiothoracic Surgery
Weill Cornell Medical College
New York, New York
March 2004

ACKNOWLEDGMENTS

This book is the result of doctors who know how to heal; Pat Piper who knows how to write these stories; editor-in-chief Tami Booth, development editor Amy Kovalski, and project editor Lois Hazel of Rodale who put their hearts and expertise into each of these pages; Spotlight Health, which made the arrangements to bring all of us together; and the assistance of my attorney and friend Mark Barondess.

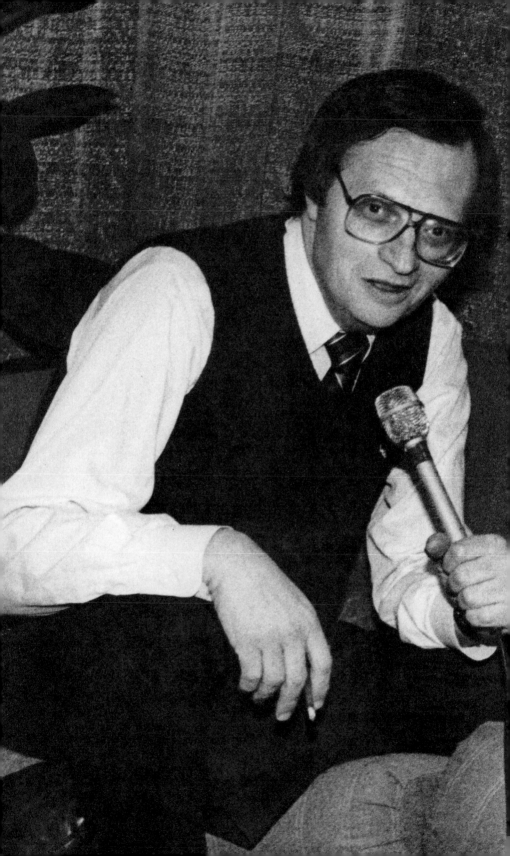

PART ONE

Early Warning Signs and Risk Factors

"Coming events cast their shadows before."

—**Thomas Campbell,**
Lochiel's Warning

February 24, 1987

I had never spent much time thinking about my heart. But when I did, it was always the other heart—the romantic one. So let's get to it right here in the first paragraph: Not paying attention to the heart (the one inside your chest) and the warnings it will send is a theme in the pages to come.

I always believed that heart attacks happened to other people. If I ever did witness one or think about one, it came to me from a television or movie screen. Redd Foxx had the best heart attack in *Sanford and Son* when he put both hands on his chest, fell into his chair, gasped for breath, and said, "This is it! This is the big one! I'm coming to you, Elizabeth!" He was fine at the end of the show because, well, he had faked the whole thing. Besides, he couldn't die because it was a hit show and he had to be back for another episode the following week. I also remember when Marlon Brando walked with his grandchild through a vegetable garden in *The Godfa-*

ther, and suddenly he, too, became short of breath, clutched his chest, and collapsed (unlike Redd Foxx, Brando's character had a real heart attack). Before this, there were all those black and white movies where the hero would lean against a wall, fist pressed against his shirt, and say to a beautiful woman, "That's okay, baby, go ahead, I'll catch up." Then he'd stagger a few feet before falling to his knees and dying—just as the violins started playing.

Those are the "Hollywood Heart Attacks." They look good on a television or movie screen, but they don't accurately portray what happens in the real world. Instead, most true-life heart attacks are a lot more low-key. But I'll tell you this: While not as dramatic as what Hollywood produces, the low-key ones get your attention pretty damn fast when they happen to you. And like the drama on the screen, everyone figures a heart attack—or any type of heart problem, for that matter—always happens to someone else. I never thought about it any more than that, which presumes that I even thought about it at all.

In early 1987 I was smoking three packs of Nat Sherman cigarettes a day, eating fried this-and-that, enjoying lamb chops with lots of fat because that always improves the taste, ordering banana cream or lemon meringue pie for dessert—and feeling absolutely fine. But when I look back at the events leading up to that day when you-know-what happened, I remember people giving me "the look." It was always followed by something like "Larry, you oughta (fill in the blank: stop smoking/eat more fish/get some exercise)," and I always responded with a completely phony appreciative nod and continued doing what I was doing. I guess that line about "everything you need to see is always right in front of you but you gotta open your eyes to see it" really does hold true. But if you don't see it, well, that's why so many people are a part of this book.

On the night before "It" happened, America's chief doctor, Surgeon General C. Everett Koop, leaned over to me after an interview on television and said, "Larry, you don't look very good." I changed the subject, made small talk, said good-bye at the studio door, and forgot about it. But later, during my late-night radio show, my right shoulder really started aching. The guest that night was author David Halberstam, who leaned over to me after the hour and said, "Larry, you don't . . . ."

You know what he said.

The pain stayed with me through the night. In the early morning, after a fitful off-and-on sleep, I woke and realized it wasn't my shoulder that was hurting now, but my stomach. I called a cardiologist I had seen in Baltimore who said that it might be a gallbladder problem, but whatever it is, I should get to a hospital sooner rather than later. It was 8:00 A.M. and I had reached the point where I knew something was wrong. Not once did it ever occur to me, though, that I was actually having a heart attack. Whatever was happening, I figured it was probably my stomach and would, no doubt, be something for which I could get a pill or an injection and be back home in no time at all. Yeah, I know.

I called my television producer, Tammy Haddad, and said, "I think I need to go to the hospital." Then I gulped down some Maalox, thinking it might help a bad stomach or a bad gallbladder. Within a few minutes, Tammy was downstairs to take me to the emergency room at George Washington University Hospital. As we crossed the Potomac River on the Memorial Bridge en route to the hospital, I lit the always-necessary cigarette.

By the time we arrived, the pain was gone.

"The hell with it," I said. "Let's go back. I'm fine." Tammy, who has never been known for her quiet ways or meekness, suggested otherwise. But I told her if there was a line, I wasn't going to wait and I'd be right out.

Well, there was a line. So I did a 180 and, true to my word, came back out the door, where a cop was telling Tammy she couldn't park in the driveway because this is where ambulances pull up. I was about to let her know I was back and we could leave when she pulled away. In keeping with my Type A view of life, I turned around and went back in, expecting to find a way to avoid the damn line, while Tammy found a parking spot somewhere on M Street.

I wasn't there for more than a minute before a young Black guy in a green hospital coat came up to me and asked if I was feeling okay. I fought back the inclination to say, "Look, I'm standing in an ER on a Tuesday morning when I could be at home. How do you think I'm feeling?" Then he moved in closer and looked right at me. "Are you a cardiac patient?"

I thought of all the people ahead of me and figured that if you're a cardiac patient, you must get into something like the express checkout lane at the grocery store (okay, "checkout" is the wrong word). Besides, the doctor I had called in Baltimore was a cardiologist, so it wasn't a complete lie. I told the guy I was.

"Let's go," he said, and we went through a set of double

doors, where a bunch of men and women in blue coats and green coats and white coats were working on patients. I was placed on a table, wires were hooked to my chest and arms and legs, a blood pressure monitor was put on one arm, a blood oxygen monitor was put on one finger, blood was taken from an artery, I was given oxygen and asked about 20 questions regarding allergies/name/who should be called/what I was feeling and where I was feeling it—to name just a few things that occurred all at once.

One of the ER physicians, Dr. Warren Levy, stood over me, looked at the results from the tests that had been taken so far, and said, "I don't like how you look," an observation I was really getting tired of hearing. I wasn't feeling any pain and told him so, but he suggested we wait 30 minutes or so to see if the symptoms returned. By this time, Tammy was in the emergency room with me, as was my radio producer. I figured, "Well, the morning is shot anyway, and maybe I can be out of here in time to make my lunch appointment at Duke Zeibert's downtown." They took an EKG and reviewed the page with the blood gases (a measurement of oxygen and other things in the blood I can't pronounce) that had been taken from the catheter in my arm.

Suddenly, I felt my right shoulder tighten. I nodded to Dr. Levy, who had been joined by another cardiologist working in the ER that day, Dr. Richard Katz. They did another EKG and the results were placed on a lighted board across the room. Again, they checked the new measurements of my blood gases. Lying on the gurney, I could see them point between the two pages and then, as if on cue, they turned at the same time to look at me. "This ain't gonna be good," I said as they both started heading in my direction.

"Mr. King," Dr. Levy said, "there is only one way to tell you this. You're having a heart attack and you're having it this minute." Even though I was lying down, the words knocked me off my feet. I've heard them every day since that February morning. It's as though someone took out The Sledge Hammer of Reality and swung it right into my face, knocking me down and sending 54 years of denial and illusion into the air. Now, only the real me was left, and I was facing the real truth. My mind was going 100 miles an hour. To me I said, "You've been fooling yourself and you didn't see it." To the doctors who were standing on either side of the gurney, I asked, "Am I going to die?"

"You're in the best place to have a heart attack," Dr. Levy assured me, "and you got here quickly." As he spoke, I wasn't taking any of the good news in. I was in an emergency room and I couldn't get past the idea that everyone is there because of bad news. I was scared.

"There's another thing," Dr. Levy said. He was bending down as he spoke. "We are one of 25 hospitals in the United States using an experimental drug called tPA." I think he started to explain what the hell tPA stood for, but I couldn't have cared less about the 25-syllable words he used. What I do remember was him saying it had yet to be approved by the Food and Drug Administration and, as a result, he was going to have to read something and read it fast because if tPA was going to be given to me and if it was going to work, it was going to have to be

TIME IS MUSCLE

Of the 1.2 million heart attacks that occur every year, more than 460,000 are fatal. Fifty percent of the fatal heart attacks are the result of a simple fact—the patient didn't get to a hospital within an hour of the first symptom. According to the National Heart, Lung, and Blood Institute, most Americans wait on average from 2 to 6 hours after the onset of heart attack symptoms before calling for help. (Women, especially, tend to delay calling 9-1-1. Most physicians believe this is, in part, because women have a higher pain threshold than men do as well as more subtle symptoms.) When you consider that a heart attack does the most damage to the heart muscle during the first 2 hours, you can see why getting medical care as soon as possible is crucial.

Further, many people ask a friend or loved one to drive them to the hospital instead of calling an ambulance, and this decision can be deadly. Today, Emergency Medical Technicians (EMTs) and paramedics are trained to treat a heart attack while en route to the emergency room. In addition, they are in contact with the hospital and can provide essential information during transport rather than having the emergency room physicians obtain the data upon arrival. This results in quicker treatment and increases the patient's chances of survival.

done as soon as possible. All I got from that conversation was that tPA would break the blood clot that was causing the heart attack. So as soon as he was done with the spiel, a clipboard with a single typed page was placed in front of me. After I signed it, a witness added his signature and tPA started flowing into my bloodstream. Within 5 minutes, the pain disappeared. Today, administering tPA to people having heart attacks is standard procedure in a hospital emergency room. Yeah, I'm one of the trailblazers. Columbus sailed the Atlantic. Lewis and Clark crossed the country. I took tPA. Same thing.

The fact of the matter was I had plenty of warning signs that my heart was in trouble (as it turned out, the inferior—obviously an appropriate name—wall of the left ventricle wasn't getting enough blood). Most heart attack patients have some indication that something isn't right. Six years earlier I had been walking to the New York Hilton from—where else—Nat Sherman's Tobacconist when my chest felt heavy. I stopped for a minute along Sixth Avenue to take a rest, and the pain went away. But as soon as I started walking again, the pressure returned to my chest. By the time I got back to my room at the Hilton, I canceled all the appointments and meetings that had been scheduled, preferring to just lie down and take it easy.

When I returned to Washington, I went to George Washington University Hospital (the same place where I was right now) for a checkup, and that's when I first learned I had heart disease. An angiogram (a picture of the heart's blood vessels and arteries that is taken with x-rays after dye is injected into the arteries through a catheter that is threaded up through the body) revealed I had one artery that was more than 75 percent blocked, another in trouble, and a third in pretty good shape. My doctors suggested I take a stress test every 6 months and give serious thought to changing my lifestyle (quit the cigarettes, get more exercise, eat better, blah-blah-blah). I was also told to take a nitroglycerin tablet called Nitrostat whenever I felt chest pain.

The nephew of one of my boyhood friends, Herbie Cohen, was Dr. David Blumenthal, a New York–based cardiologist who looked at my tests and recommended a Baltimore cardiologist for me to see for the follow-up tests and exams. That was the guy I had called earlier that morning.

When a doctor asked me during my earlier checkup about heart disease in my family, I remember the concern on his face when I said my father had died of it at age 43. Did any of this sink in? Let me put it this way: I left the doctor's office thinking my dad died a long time ago when medicine wasn't as good as it is now. In fact, I lit a cigarette thinking about it.

Yes, the word "denial" is appropriate here.

Dr. Levy and Dr. Katz were now standing over me saying the heart attack had passed, but they wanted to keep me in the hospital for a few days. My daughter Chaia was at my side, and I remember telling her to get in touch with my agent, Bob Woolf, and let him know what had happened and where I was. Suddenly, a lot of things had to be done: Replacements needed to be found for my CNN show; a substitute host had to located for my Mutual Broadcasting System radio show; affiliates had to be contacted before news got out about what had happened. Most of all, some sense of "everything's under control" had to be maintained even though, from my perspective, nothing was under control—and if it was, certainly nothing was going to be the same ever again.

The young man who had brought me into the ER was now at my side, and I learned he was assigned to look for people coming in who were pallid and pale—just one sign of a heart attack about to happen. Looking back, I guess I was pale, hence all the comments for the past 24 hours. "Son of a bitch," I thought to myself as they wheeled me down a hall, "it has happened to me."

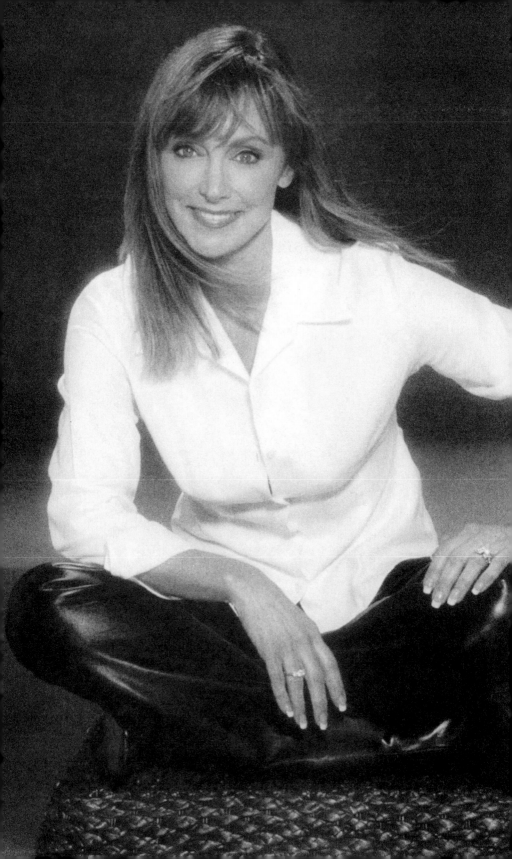

PEGGY FLEMING

At the 1968 Winter Olympics, Peggy Fleming skated away with a gold medal— and elegantly capped off 5 years of being an American figure skating champion. Only 19 years old, she had already dominated world-level women's skating competitions. In 1981, Peggy moved from the rink to the broadcast booth to analyze skating events for ABC Sports. Based on her achievements, Sports Illustrated *named Peggy Fleming as one of the seven athletes who changed the game in the 20th century. She lives with her husband and one of her two sons in the San Francisco Bay area, where they make wine from grapes in their vineyard. (Her other son lives in Colorado with his wife and two sons.) Today, Peggy is an advocate for knowing the risk factors of heart disease because she has two of them: a family history of heart troubles and high cholesterol.*

"Even though I may have to work a little harder at it now, I'm determined to stay healthy and beat the odds for someone with my family history."

Some years ago, I was talking to a cardiologist who is a friend of the family and somehow we got on the subject of cholesterol. He looked at my son Andy, who was about to go off to college. "You know," he said to me, "he should be tested." The doctor was aware that my father had died of a heart attack at 41, while I was preparing to skate in the Olympics. Because of my family history, I knew the importance of keeping an eye on cholesterol levels. So we went to his office, and both my son and I had stress tests and cholesterol screenings done. The results showed that everything was fine, but I was told that this is something we needed to watch.

This brief trip to the doctor was the first time I had taken an active role in paying attention to my risk factors for heart disease. I sent Andy off to college with a total cholesterol of 165 or something like that (well under the 200 level at which doctors start to worry). My own cholesterol level was 194—still considered normal—and so we weren't concerned. This was 1996.

Heart Disease Strikes Close to Home

In 2000, my younger sister, Maxine (who was just 50 years old), suddenly had a heart attack and died, leaving two children ages 13 and 16. This started the red flags coming up for me. And it was Maxine's death that took me back to the doctor to have my cholesterol doublechecked. It had gone up to 234. Since my family history wasn't very good with cholesterol, my doctor prescribed cholesterol-lowering medication. He believed that even though I was exercising and eating right, my genetic history put me at risk.

I have another sister who went through triple bypass surgery in 2001. She was only 47. I had pushed her to go in and get a checkup. She wasn't going to go, and she was a nurse! She was trying to diagnose herself. She would say, "I know I need to stop smoking and lose some weight," but she didn't really get anywhere with it.

She and I had gone for a walk, and she was having chest pains, though we weren't even walking that fast. I said, "Cathy, this is not normal." What was frustrating was that her doctor at the time would say, "Well, don't walk so fast." When I heard that, I said, "That can't be right." I urged her to go in for another test, and when she did, they wouldn't let her come home. They scheduled surgery for the very next day. After the surgery, she said, "Oh my God, why didn't I listen to you all these years?"

I've come to learn I can do only so much. Why didn't Maxine listen to me? Cathy is a different person now. She's lost more than 60 pounds. She will never smoke again. And she's really careful about what she eats. She was scared to death when she was told she needed bypass surgery. She had never had any surgery before, and this surgery is as big as it gets. Before the operation, she'd tell me, "I just can't do this." I remember telling her, "You have every right to be scared, but you have to do this. When you're faced with something that you absolutely have to do, you'll do it and you'll find out you're stronger than you think you are."

Back when I was skating, I'd hear the words "high cholesterol," but it was always about my dad who died in 1966. He was supposed to watch his diet; he had had two heart attacks before the third one that killed him. Our family breakfasts back then were always a lot of bacon and eggs. My father would say, "I'm going to live my life the way I want to live it," and you know, that's okay. We can't dictate how other people should live. It is their life, and we can't look down on them because they're not doing what we'd hoped. Still, I think it's selfish of a person to say, "Who cares?" There are a lot of people who care.

My younger sister did the same thing. She didn't go to the doctor regularly, she smoked, she was overweight, and she knew she had lots of risk factors, but she just didn't want to think about them. And she was an intelligent, college-educated young woman. She was happy, and that's the way she wanted to live her life. After she passed away, we had trouble coming to grips with that: Why didn't she go to the doctor? Why didn't we urge her to stop smoking? Why didn't we do more? Well, we tried, but it would always end up in an argument. It hurts. It's so hard for the people who are left behind—they're the ones who really suffer.

Fighting Back

Today, I'm much more aware of what I'm eating. I had a really good diet when I was skating. My mom was on the cutting edge back then: She served me meals with high protein, low carbs, no dessert—well, okay, dessert once in a while, but no soda pop. We had juices and waters. When I was competing, there were times when I couldn't even get down a meal because of my nerves. But my mom knew I loved macaroni and cheese, so she'd make that before an event and it was perfect.

I see food as fuel. I believe that if you eat the right things, you'll have more energy and you'll look and feel better. When I go to a restaurant, I try to stay away from the bread and butter. And pastas with cream sauces are just deadly. They taste wonderful, but they're so high in fat. I'll order a small serving of rice—maybe a quarter of a cup—instead of getting the huge portions typically served. Along with that, I'll order a small portion—or a couple of appetizers—of something else, so I have a variety of small portions rather than a single huge portion. It works.

I think the fast-food places are trying to be better. If I have to go to one, I'll eat only half of the bread and take the hamburger or grilled chicken—I don't order the breaded chicken—and eat the lettuce and tomatoes and have no sauce at all. The tomato really makes it juicy. Just don't order the fries. They've got salads now, too. I hope in 10 years it will be healthy to go to a fast-food restaurant. When I travel, I bring protein bars or walnuts, which have zero cholesterol and lots of protein and good carbs. I have that instead of cholesterol-filled potato chips.

When I go grocery shopping, I read labels. I try to avoid trans fats as much as possible; they're in all kinds of packaged foods. I stay with the fresh stuff—there are fewer labels to read!

Recently, my son came to visit for Thanksgiving and he had started putting on weight. He's a big snowboarder, and he was eating a lot of fast food. I was scheduled to get some bloodwork done anyway, so I insisted that he come with me and I would pay for his bloodwork. His cholesterol was over 200. I remember the shocked look on his face when he saw the results.

I took him to the cardiologist, who said, "Let's first see if we can correct this with diet." That works for him. He's only 26. It was a wake-up call, though, and he got really scared—look at his genetics, wow. Sometimes you just have to follow your intuition, and I'm glad I had him have that bloodwork. It just goes to prove that you may be young and you may look healthy, but cholesterol isn't something that you can see. You have to be tested for it. You don't feel it. It's a silent killer.

I think when it comes to preventing heart disease, you must develop strategies that work for you as an individual. We are all a little different, and each person's body chemistry works differently as well, so what works for one person may not work for somebody else. Given my experience, I believe you need to sit down with your doctor and evaluate your personal health and risk factors, including your physical makeup, diet, exercise program, and family history. Ask him or her to work with you so that together, you can create a personalized plan of action.

For example, estrogen is a good cholesterol fighter. Now that I'm 55, my estrogen levels are decreasing. That's why my cholesterol started shooting up. I'm getting older and my body is changing, and what used to work in my thirties doesn't work in my fifties. Yet even though I may have to work a little harder at it now, I'm determined to stay healthy and beat the odds for someone with my family history. And I'm confident that my son will, too.

Factoring In the Risks

When it comes to heart disease, at least we know where we stand. Thanks to a study conducted in 2003 by The Cleveland Clinic Heart Center, there is now no question about the major risk factors for developing the nation's number one killer. The combined study of several trials involved a total of 122,458 patients with coronary artery disease (heart attack and angioplasty). The ranges in this study revealed that between 80 and 90 percent of the patients had at least one major risk factor (high cholesterol, high blood pressure, diabetes, or smoking). Prior to this finding, doctors believed that risk factors were absent in at least half of all the patients with coronary artery disease. The good news is that lifestyle plays a role in most of the risk factors, which means that they are preventable. Here are the main enemies in the fight against heart disease:

High cholesterol. One out of every two Americans is believed to have high cholesterol. If you haven't already, visit your doctor for a lipid profile, which measures your total cholesterol, LDL and HDL cholesterol, and triglycerides. You'll need to fast for 9 to 12 hours before the blood sample is drawn. LDL clogs your arteries; a reading of 100 to 129 mg/dL (milligrams per deciliter) is considered near optimal. For LDL, the lower the number, the better. On the other hand, HDL escorts LDL out of the body and helps to keep your arteries clean, so a higher number is better. In men, HDL should be greater than 40; in women, it should be greater than 50. To get your total cholesterol number, add your LDL and HDL together. Less than 200 is desirable. Numbers between 201 and 239 are considered borderline high, while a reading above 240 means you have twice the risk of heart disease as a person with a total cholesterol of 200. For triglycerides, less than 150 mg/dL is considered normal.

High blood pressure. "Blood pressure" refers to the force of blood against the walls of the arteries. It is measured with two numbers: the systolic, which is always the first number and measures the force of blood when the heart is pumping, and the diastolic, which is the second number and measures the force of blood against an artery wall when the heart has contracted and isn't pushing blood through veins and arteries. You have high blood pressure if your reading is 140/90 mmHg (millimeters of mercury) or higher. Normal blood pressure is 120/80 mmHg, but it is important to realize that blood pressure will increase after age 50. High blood pressure means your heart is working harder to move blood through your body. Studies have shown that every 10-point increase in systolic blood pressure (the first number) results in a 20 percent increase in the risk for developing cardiovascular disease.

Diabetes. Two-thirds of people with diabetes die from heart disease or stroke, according to the American Diabetes Association. High blood sugar levels (150 and above) can cause blood vessels and arteries to narrow. Diabetes also increases the tendency of blood to clot and decreases the body's natural ability to dissolve clots.

Smoking. Cigarette smoke contains 4,000 different chemicals. This fact alone is enough to explain why smoking is dangerous. If you can quit for 1 year, your chance of having a heart attack is one-half that of a person who currently smokes. After 15 years of not smoking, your heart will be as healthy as that of a person who never smoked.

A high-fat diet. A diet high in saturated fats, which are found mainly in meat and dairy products, increases heart disease risk. To lower your risk, choose a diet that gets 30 percent or less of its overall calories from fat, recommends Bill Ricks, M.D., of The Heart Associates of Northern California, and Peggy Fleming's cardiologist. Remember, too, that not all fats are created equal. Instead of saturated fats like butter and margarine, choose monounsaturated fats such as olive oil and safflower oil. Doctors also recommend eating one or two 3-ounce servings of fatty fish each week. Good choices include herring, salmon, tuna, and mackerel, which contain omega-3 fatty acids that prevent the formation of blood clots. Further, the typical American diet is woefully low on fiber. Soluble fiber forms a gel that binds with cholesterol, escorting it out of the body. Doctors recommend consuming at least 25 grams of fiber a day, which you can achieve by eating plenty of fresh fruits, vegetables, grains, and legumes.

Inactivity. A sedentary lifestyle increases heart disease risk. Doctors recommend getting a minimum of 20 minutes of exercise every other day. Simply taking a brisk walk will fill the requirement; your goal is to get your heart rate to more than 100 beats per minute for the duration. (If you've been inactive, first get your doctor's okay before trying anything more strenuous than walking.)

Obesity. Research has found that men with a waist larger than 40 inches have an increased risk of heart disease. Women with a waist larger than 35 inches are also at risk.

FAST FACTS: WOMEN AND HEART DISEASE

If you think women don't need to worry about heart disease, think again. These sobering statistics come from the National Coalition for Women with Heart Disease:

◆ 8 million American women are living with heart disease.

◆ 13 percent of women age 45 and over have had a heart attack. 435,000 women have heart attacks each year, and 267,000 of these are fatal.

◆ Average age when a heart attack occurs in women: 70.4.

◆ Approximately 31,800 women die each year of congestive heart failure (the inability of the heart to pump enough blood through the arteries). That's nearly 63 percent of all deaths from congestive heart failure.

◆ African-American women ages 55 to 64 are twice as likely as White women their age to have a heart attack.

◆ Women who smoke are at risk of having a heart attack 19 years earlier than women who don't smoke.

◆ Women with diabetes are two to three times more likely to have a heart attack than women who are not diabetic.

◆ More women than men die each year of heart disease, yet women receive only 33 percent of all angioplasties, stents, and bypass surgeries; 28 percent of implantable defibrillators; and 36 percent of all open-heart surgeries.

Family history. Your risk for developing heart disease increases if you have a first-degree family member (a brother, sister, mother, or father) who has heart trouble. While you can't control your family history, you should take special care to avoid other risk factors if your family history increases your odds for developing heart disease.

Stress. High levels of stress can play a role in heart disease. For instance, cholesterol levels for accountants tend to peak during tax time, and doctors can actually tell whether their patients are personal or corporate accountants because their cholesterol levels will peak at different times of the year, reports Dr. Ricks. While other factors may have a more direct impact on whether or not someone develops heart disease, it's wise to be aware of those times in your life when you feel particularly stressed, and to make a special effort to set aside time then for meditation, yoga, or other calming activities.

MIKE WALLACE

One of the country's best-known reporters, Mike Wallace began his career on the radio in the late 1940s and moved into hosting television programs 10 years later. He was a war correspondent for CBS during the conflict in Viet Nam, and in 1968 joined a new show called 60 Minutes. *He's still there, and despite having a pacemaker implanted more than 10 years ago to regulate his heartbeat (though some who have been interviewed by him would challenge the idea he even has a heart), Mike shows no indication whatsoever that he'll step down and go slower.*

"My pacemaker hasn't stopped me from doing a thing. . . . It's a fairly easy operation, and the pacemaker has allowed me to live my life with few interruptions."

It was 1991 and I'd been having what amounted to fainting spells. I didn't know what the dickens it was all about, but I'd suddenly get dizzy. I wouldn't really faint, but I'd lie down on the couch in my office and wait for the lightheadedness to pass. But it kept happening, and every time it did, I figured, "Well, this will pass." This had been going on for about 6 months, and I kept thinking, "Well, I must be tired" or "Gee, I've got so many more important things to do right now." I never gave a lot of thought about going to see a doctor about it.

One day, I was out in California with Don Hewitt, the executive producer of *60 Minutes*. When I got on a plane for the flight back to New York, I leaned over to get something out of my bag before we took off. That was the last thing I remember. I'm told I hit the floor. I was out cold.

When Hewitt saw me go down, his reaction, I later learned, was "Damn, now we'll never be able to catch *Cheers!*" (We were in a ratings battle with the show.) They brought a stretcher on board and took me off to a Marina del Rey hospital. When I came to, I remember being given some pills while the doctors ran some tests. Finally, a doctor came with the results in his hand and said, "You need a pacemaker." That was the first time I'd ever thought about it.

The next day, I got back on a plane and flew home and went to see my cardiologist, Dr. Jeffrey Matos, in Manhattan. He did some tests and agreed with the first diagnosis—I needed a pacemaker.

I interview people for a living, so I started asking questions. I think whenever you're considering a medical procedure, you need to get informed, and that means not being afraid to ask your doctor for the information you need. I asked him, "How long am I going to be out of action? What is this going to involve? How serious is this operation? What will happen if I don't have the operation?" I play tennis, so I asked how soon after the operation I would be able to play. Sure I was apprehensive, but I also kept saying to myself, "Okay, I have to do it; this has to be done." My doctor told me there was no advantage whatsoever to waiting, and when I look back, truly, it was a minimal rearrangement of my life.

I knew people who had pacemakers. Two or three of them said, "Forget it, this is an easy operation. You won't be out of action for long at all." Frank Field, who at the time was the best-known weatherman on television in New York, told me about his experience and said, "It's a piece of cake." So within 2 weeks of being told about the device and how my life would improve, I had a new pacemaker. I was 72.

When I woke up after the surgery, my arm was hurting.

They had put it out to the left on a board and stretched it so they could more easily make the incision above my collarbone. I had muscle pain for 2 to 3 months, and I was told not to try to reach up and lift things for a few weeks. But I was back at work 10 days later, though not at full speed. And soon after that, I was back on the tennis court.

Moving On with a Pacemaker

I'm now on my second pacemaker: I had the original one replaced about a year ago because its battery had reached the end of its useful life. The new pacemaker was placed in the same incision as the original. The doctors checked out the old wires and determined they were okay, so all that was new was the pacemaker (which includes a new hermetically sealed battery).

My pacemaker hasn't stopped me from doing a thing. The only issue I face comes at airports. Whenever I'm in line for the machine that scans for metal objects, I have to tell them I have a pacemaker. They have folks with pacemakers go into a special entrance, where they pat you down. International travel has presented more of a problem; there have been a few instances when the foreign security people didn't understand why I couldn't go through their metal detectors.

Every few months, the doctor's office will call me to make sure my pacemaker is working properly. I'll place a transmitter over the spot where my pacemaker is located, and it sends a recording of my heart tracing over the phone. This is how they can tell if the pacemaker is properly stimulating my heart and if the battery is still good.

I also see my doctor every few months, and occasionally, he makes me wear a Holter monitor for 24 hours. It records my heart rhythm as I go about my day and is another way to make sure my pacemaker is working properly. The monitor gives him detailed information that a regular pacemaker can't.

For 10 to 15 years prior to the surgery, I had tried to give up smoking. I would give it up, then fall off the wagon, then give it up again, then fall off again, and so on. But I haven't had a cigarette since that operation, that's for damn sure. Before the pacemaker, I had quit in my mind, but I was obviously still hooked. I kept saying, "Well, I've really minimized the amount of smoking I do now." But the day I walked out of the hospital, I said, "Okay, now I'm sure as hell not going to smoke."

I've always been fairly sensible about my diet, and I haven't changed it much since that day I got on the airplane with Don Hewitt. I was married for 28 years to a woman who fed me mainly nuts and raisins. She wasn't a health nut, but she was ahead of her time. We had a lot of fish and a lot of chicken without the skin. I did ask Dr. Matos about my diet, but he told me there is nothing about having a pacemaker that is a determinant about what I can and can't eat. Obviously, like everyone else, I still need to eat a healthful diet, but diet isn't as much a concern for me as it is for someone who had a bypass or angioplasty.

To anyone facing this surgery, I say, "Go do it." Although there are always risks, it's a fairly easy operation, and the pacemaker has allowed me to live my life with few interruptions. And it certainly beats passing out on a plane!

⌒

The Doctor's Notes:
ACCELERATING A SLOW HEART RATE

JEFFREY MATOS, M.D., president of
Arrhythmia Associates of New York, based in New York City

On average, the human heart beats about 70 times per minute when we're at rest. In order to maintain this rate, three structures in the heart—the sinus node, the AV node, and the His-Purkinje system—must all function properly. The sinus node is the heart's natural pacemaker. It stimulates the heart with a tiny electric current. The AV node and the His-Purkinje system are internal "wires" that allow an electric link between the top two chambers of the heart (the atria, which are the minor pumping chambers) and the bottom two chambers (the ventricles, which are the major pumping chambers). These three are the natural determinants of the heart rate, and when any one of these components malfunctions, the heart may slow down to a dangerous rate.

To speed up a slow heart rate, doctors may install an artificial pacemaker, which is a small, battery-operated device that helps the heart beat in a regular rhythm.

In Mike Wallace's case, the His-Purkinje system wasn't up to par. Each of the other structures worked properly, so it was reasonable to conclude that a problem in the His-Purkinje system was the reason he was losing consciousness. His heart wasn't beating fast enough to get blood and oxygen to his brain, which is why he lost consciousness.

When I'm asked what the risks of pacemakers are, I say there's a risk of infection by implanting the device. Even though it's done in operating room conditions, any foreign object can get infected. So we discuss that. The patient will need to receive antibiotics before and after the pacemaker is inserted. There's also a risk of bleeding. For example, on rare occasions, the pacemaker wire may poke a hole in the heart. There's also a small risk that the pacemaker could have a technical defect, or that a lung or arm problem may result.

Prior to the procedure, patients will get intravenous sedation, so they are kind of groggy. We avoid "general anesthesia" because the deeper you put somebody out, the riskier the procedure becomes for anesthesia-related reasons. Pacemakers are generally put in a little bit below the collarbone, typically on the left side. If, however, the patient is left-handed or there is some sort of technical difficulty with the left side, the pacemaker can be placed on the right side. The procedure usually takes less than an hour. ▪

Living with a Pacemaker

Most patients find that a pacemaker has very little impact on their lives. For the first 6 weeks after having a pacemaker implanted, it's important to limit how much you lift your arms above your head. This doesn't mean you can't get something off the top shelf of your closet, but you should refrain from activities like golf and tennis. This is because it takes about 6 weeks for a meshwork of heart fibers to grow over the lead (or leads) that run from the pacemaker to the heart, forming a natural "glue." Before that time, excessive activity can cause a lead to move out of place.

Over the long term, the pacemaker wires are subject to a certain amount of "wear and tear." They may be damaged at the point where they pass under the collarbone. Furthermore, the heart beats about 70 times a minute; that's more than 100,000 times a day and more than 35 million times in a year. And every time it beats, the wires bend slightly.

There is one other patient restriction, and this one is permanent: People with pacemakers cannot have MRI (Magnetic Resonance Imaging) or MRA (Magnetic Resonance Angiography) tests. The magnetic field that patients are exposed to during these tests can affect the pacemaker, damaging it, and making it act inappropriately.

Eventually, a pacemaker will need to be replaced. How long a patient can go before this becomes necessary depends on a number of factors. One of the main issues is how often it's used.

Since pacemakers kick in only when necessary, some people's pacemakers may be in use much more often than others. Like any other battery-operated device, the more it's used, the more quickly it will need to be replaced. And, like a flashlight, if you hardly use it, the batteries still aren't going to last forever. The average battery life is about 7 years, but there are people who will go through batteries in 3 or 4 years, while others will make 10 or 11 years. When you replace it, you literally take the old pacemaker out; you can't just change the batteries because they are sealed inside the pacemaker. The procedure takes about 40 minutes and sometimes requires an overnight stay in a hospital.

Patients with pacemakers can have them checked two different ways: with a telephone that transmits about 10 seconds of the pacemaker's activity and tells the doctor some rudimentary things about the functioning of the pacemaker, or during an office visit. This is where an interrogation is done to determine details of the battery status, the status of the wires that connect the pacemaker to the heart, and more general information about what the heart rhythm has been in a broad sense. The information obtained during the office interrogation is more detailed than that obtained during a telephone check.

—JEFFREY MATOS, M.D., *president of Arrhythmia Associates of New York, based in New York City*

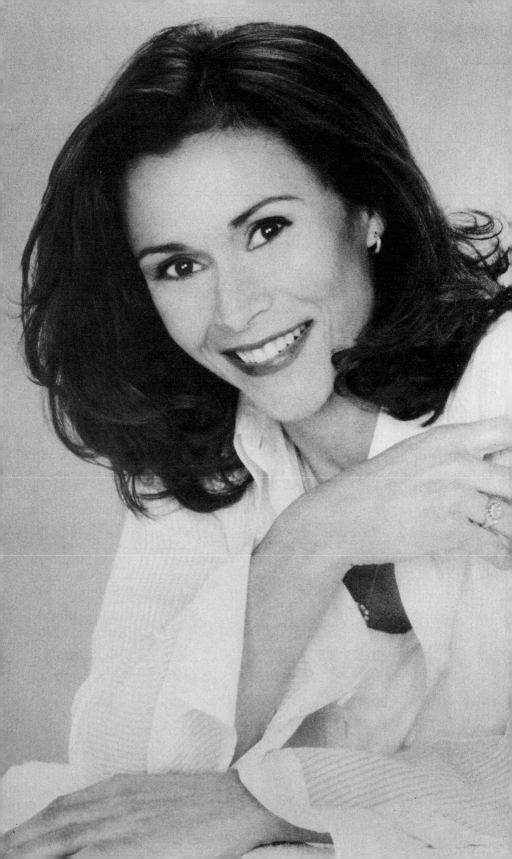

KATE JACKSON

First seen in ABC's Dark Shadows
(1966–71), Kate Jackson went on to star in
Charlie's Angels *(1976–81) and CBS's*
Scarecrow and Mrs. King *(1983–87). Al-*
ready a breast cancer survivor, she was diag-
nosed at age 46 with a hole in her heart.
The news came as a complete surprise, and
it changed her life forever. Yet despite
having heart surgery, this award-winning
actress has stayed in motion. Today, she
makes made-for-television movies through
her own production company.

"After undergoing heart surgery, I've learned not to get stressed out over business anymore. I can laugh about it. I know what my priorities are."

In 1994, I wrapped up a television movie in North Carolina called *Justice in a Small Town* and decided to visit my mom in Alabama on the way back to California. At the time, I knew something wasn't right with my health because while we were filming the movie, I was feeling absolutely fatigued and I was aware that my heart would beat much faster than normal when I had to exert energy. For example, in one scene I had to carry a very light little girl and run through our trailer home on the set, and we had to do the shot three times. I just had to run inside, run through the trailer, grab stuff while carrying her, and run out. We did it the first time and I was breathing kind of heavily afterward. We did it a second time and I was breathing harder. Before we started the third take, I was standing outside the door waiting for action and my heart was beating so hard. The little girl was moving in my arms, going back and forth from my chest because my heart was beating so loudly. She looked at me and I knew why. I said, "Boy, my heart sure beats hard, doesn't it?" and she said yes and looked at me. And then we did the shot a third time and I remember thinking afterward, "Good Lord, I hope they got it because I'm really out of breath."

The last 2 weeks of the shoot we were doing day-for-nights, so the grips put really heavy black material over the bedroom windows in our hotel suites so it was as black as night and I could easily sleep from 5:00 or 6:00 in the morning until 2:00 in the afternoon. But I knew that when I got to Alabama, it was going to be really hard to adjust my body clock back to regular daytime hours. It's worse than jet lag, and I figured okay, I'll probably have a couple of bad days, but I'll be all right. So I didn't sleep the first night I arrived in Alabama, and then the bulldozers started working on a new house next door. I ended up going sleepless for 3 nights, and I could feel myself starting to lose it. I was just so tired and I'd start crying.

For some time, I had also noticed that my skin had a bluish tint to it. While I was doing the movie, my hair and makeup people noticed it and were worried something might be wrong, but they didn't say anything to me. When I saw it, I attributed it to the lighting in the area where the makeup artists worked, and thought maybe it was set for daytime when it should have been set for nighttime. When I was in Alabama, I could still see the blue tint in my face, but I figured it must be the light in the bathroom. Well, after 3 days of feeling so horrible, I had to do something. I had hit the wall.

I called Dr. Jerry Pohost and said, "I think I need to go to the hospital." I knew him because he had done an angioplasty on my mother. He picked me up, got me a hospital room, and ordered some tests. We talked about what we would say was the matter so some big story wouldn't come out in the tabloids. "Let's just say dizziness," he suggested. I was going to blame exhaustion, but he said nobody could make anything out of dizziness.

A Stunning Diagnosis

I have this little movie in my mind, and I replay it now and then. I'm in my hospital room, Dr. Pohost is walking toward the door, and then he turns around and says, "Well, I am a cardiologist, so I might as well listen to your heart."

Dr. Pohost placed his stethoscope on my chest for a few moments and then walked out the door. A few minutes later, an ultrasound machine was wheeled into the room accompanied by a lot of doctors and nurses.

The next day, Dr. Pohost came back and sat in a chair to talk with me. The conversation took sort of a quirky turn and I said, "Jerry? Sounds like we're talking about heart surgery."

He looked at me and said, "Yes Kate, we are."

"Jerry, it sounds like we're talking about heart surgery for me."

And he said, "Yes Kate, we are."

So I said, "Are we talking about 20 years? 15 years?"

He said, "How about 2 weeks?"

Dr. Pohost explained that I had a hole in my heart, and the reason I was out of breath was that my body was getting only half the amount of blood (and, therefore, oxygen) it should be getting. He explained it this way: Say you have 2 quarts of oxygenated blood. Normally, all 2 quarts of blood are pumped out of the heart, delivering a rich supply of oxygen to the rest of your body. In my case, though, only 1 quart was getting pumped out and the other one would go back through the hole and get reprocessed. So I was getting only half of what I should have been getting from my heart. The hole had been there all my life, and I'm assuming that as I got older, it got larger. Jerry also explained that my skin appeared blue because the blood traveling through the hole in my heart lacked oxygen.

Well, news like that is always a shock, and I know I was surprised. But at least I finally knew why I had been feeling so tired and why I was breathing so hard. I knew something else, too: I was ready to have the surgery done.

If you're going to have any kind of heart surgery, you must believe in and trust your doctor, and you have to have a reason to do that. You must do your research. Find the best possible person to care for you. I had a little notebook with questions that I had used when looking for a cardiologist to do an angioplasty on my mother. But it was also useful for taking notes, because nobody is going to remember everything that is said, especially if you're talking about open-heart surgery. I really believe that when it comes to your health, it's your responsibility to be actively involved. I did all the research myself, most of it using the Internet. So I asked, "How many times have you performed the operation? How many times was it successful?" These are questions you want to ask whether you're considering angioplasty or the repair of a hole in your heart. If the doctor has been successful only 25 out of 100 times, that's not the person you want. And you certainly don't want to be his first patient. I knew Jerry Pohost and trusted him—and he was with me every single step of the way.

I wanted to know everything that was going to happen. I had Dr. Pohost spell it out for me if I didn't understand some-

"IT CAN'T BE HEART DISEASE . . . I'M A WOMAN!"

When it comes to heart disease, women are sometimes their own worst advocates. Particularly in the case of a heart attack, getting treatment quickly can mean the difference between life and death. Yet a look at the following facts shows that women often put off treatment or are reluctant to call an ambulance when symptoms become severe.

♦ Women are more likely than men to question their symptoms before seeking medical assistance. As a result, they may wait longer than men before seeking help.

♦ Some women delay seeking care because of domestic responsibilities (the need to finish preparing a meal or care for their spouse or children, for example) or fear of embarrassment if it's a false alarm ("What will the neighbors say if they see an ambulance in the driveway?").

thing. I asked, "And that does what?" or "And when does that happen?" I had a clear picture of what was going to go on.

I went back to California, and quite honestly, I got my affairs in order. Open-heart surgery means that your heart is going to be stopped and the doctors are going to hold it in their hands. So things that people don't like to think about need to be taken care of. I made a new will. I was living at the beach

◆ Women are more likely than men to have themselves driven by a friend or spouse to an ER, rather than calling an ambulance. But this can sometimes be a deadly mistake, since paramedics on board ambulances begin treating a heart attack immediately.

◆ Women continue to believe heart disease is a "man's disease." They have taken ownership of breast cancer and are well aware of the need to obtain an annual mammogram, but they often don't give their hearts the same high priority. While there is no single test to accurately diagnose heart disease, there are a number of tests that can help tell whether an individual is at risk for, or already has, heart disease. Women need to ask their doctors what tests are appropriate for them, whether the tests are accurate in women, and how their individual risk factors (genetics, obesity, high cholesterol, high blood pressure, smoking) should be addressed.

—SHARONNE HAYES, M.D., *director of the Mayo Women's Heart Clinic in Rochester, Minnesota*

but had just bought a new house. I talked to the designer who was helping me and explained that I was going to have surgery and would be recuperating for a month in Alabama. Then I'd come back and be in front of the camera in September. (I was already scheduled as the co-executive producer for my next television movie in 4 months. It was an action-adventure film to be shot on location in the Yukon territory in Alaska. In it, I had to play the very athletic role of a woman who races in the Iditarod dog sled event.)

I called my agent and said that this was no big deal, that the doctors found it in time, and they expected to be able to fix it. I said that I wasn't going to be handicapped in any way, and that it hadn't caused any irreparable damage. I was trying to be reassuring, because in Los Angeles, you can be crazy, you can be late to the set, or you can not know your words and hold everybody up while you learn them and the industry won't like it, but you *cannot* be sick. I thought back to a time during a shooting of an episode of *Charlie's Angels* guest-starring Ross Martin, who had done *The Wild, Wild West*. Ross had a heart attack, recovered, and was ready for more work. During shooting, he talked about how hard it was for him to get a job because people were afraid he was going to have a heart attack on the spot. It was a problem for him. I wish that we were all enlightened enough now to know that—regardless of the field of work they are in—people who have had heart surgery can go on to lead happy, healthy, and productive lives.

When you have open-heart surgery, there's that scar that runs from just below your collarbone all the way down the front of you. I thought, "Geez, if I have that scar, there isn't any chance I could even wear a button-up blouse." So I asked the doctors if they could go in through my side instead. They agreed, and had me lie on my left side. A little part of the scar is on my back and then comes under my right arm, almost to the middle of my chest—a very neat and tidy little scar. I did it that way so I would have more options in the clothes I wore on-screen. Had I not been in the profession I'm in, I don't think I would have worried about it. But I knew I was going to have to wear an evening gown, or I would be told "here's your wardrobe" and I would have to say, "I can't wear anything but turtlenecks."

I had cracked my wrist on the movie I had just finished, and one of the last things I remember in the OR was asking them to please not bend my wrist. I also remember thinking how tiny the room looked and that it didn't look anything like what I used to watch on *Ben Casey* or *Dr. Kildare* or *ER*.

I wanted to try to do two things: The first was to try to remember if I had an out-of-body experience during the operation. The second goal was more earthly: I knew when I woke up, I'd have a tube in my mouth, and I wanted to remember not to jerk on it. Well, I don't recall any out-of-body experience, so I don't believe I had one. But I did remember not to pull on the tube in my mouth when I woke up. Instead, I made a few sounds to let the nurses know I was awake, and they took the tube out. The staff had told my mom that I would be awake by 5:00 in the afternoon and she said, "Is that when normal people wake up?" They said yes and she responded, "Well, Katie will probably be awake by 11:30 or 12:00. Be watching for her."

INTENSIVE CARE — AND A CALL FROM CHER

The moment I woke up, I knew I was all right. I knew I had a perfect heart, a normal heart for the first time in my life. I told myself I was going to take care of it and take care of myself.

Knowing you have made it successfully through surgery and have a new lease on life is a wonderful feeling, despite how you are feeling physically at the moment.

In intensive care, you don't get telephone calls. But they were sort of sitting me up after the tube was taken out, and I wasn't really sure what they were trying to do. I remember thinking, "I must be hallucinating because it seems someone is trying to stretch a telephone on a long cord over to me." I kept thinking, "This can't be," but I did take the phone and it was Cher. She's probably the only person in the world who could get through to you in intensive care!

I was glad to talk to her because it got my mind on something else. Cher said, "You're all right! You're fine. You did it! You were great!" And I said, "Yeah, I always knew I'd be a fabulous heart surgeon." While I listened to Cher, I could see two doctors position themselves to my side and suddenly, they pulled out the tube that was in my upper back. As it came out, I groaned "Whoa," but I was glad to have had my attention taken away from it because I think it would have really hurt if I was focused on what they were going to do. Cher was very enthusiastic and relieved, and looking back, I know it was helpful to hear from her at that moment. I was still groggy, but Cher wanted to make sure I understood that everything was fine.

The day after surgery, I was already walking a bit, but only in my room. I was very sore and couldn't raise or lower myself very well. Lying down and getting up were hard. By the following day, I walked slowly—very slowly—down the corridor and all the way around the unit and then all the way around twice and then three or four times, all with an IV stand alongside me. I could tell the difference by the next day. I knew something was different about me and about the way I felt; my head seemed clearer. I had the operation on a Monday and was supposed to go home the following Saturday, but I decided to go home a day early. I went home to my house in Alabama, and friends came over and took walks with me. At first, I couldn't even walk a block, so we worked up to longer walks gradually. I was really committed to getting back in shape.

While my body was healing physically, I had a strange experience that was much more difficult for me to understand. There's a notorious period doctors will tell you about when people who are recovering from heart surgery get depressed. It just kind of goes with the whole event—and it *is* an event. For me, it started a few days after the surgery and ended about 2 or 3 months later. I'd be talking to somebody and all of a sudden, out of nowhere, I'd burst into tears. I would excuse myself from the room until I could calm down, but soon it started happening in business meetings for a movie I was co-producing. I'd just say, "This is nothing, it's from the heart surgery; let's continue with the meeting, please," while tears were coming down my face. "Don't pay any attention to me," I'd repeat. People got used to that. It was really very strange. I made a point of watching who I would talk to, and I also knew that at certain times of the day I'd be more teary than at others.

When I'm doing a movie, I always try to get as much sleep as I can, and I've started taking naps during the day. I tell myself "I'm tired," and try to baby myself a little bit. This isn't to say I work only 12 hours a day and that's it; although for the first two movies I did after surgery, I did write into my contract that I could work only a specific number of hours each day and no more than that. I am not, and have never been, afraid of working hard—you do what has to be done. But I will tell you, in these times and in this town, producers are making more money and giving less of it to the people who are making it for them. After undergoing heart surgery, I've learned not to get stressed out over business anymore. I can laugh about it. I know what my priorities are.

It's a sad truth that one out of every two women will die of a heart attack, stroke, or cardiovascular disease, and yet only one out of every ten women knows that fact. Heart problems are not strictly a man's disease. I encourage every woman to make a special appointment with her doctor when she reaches her 45th or 50th birthday. This is the time when male executives are routinely put on a stress test machine to get an indication of their heart health. I think women should demand the same preventive care. Say to your doctor, "Treat me as if I were a 55-year-old CEO with a wife and kids. Give my heart every test you would give that man's."

Think about it: You always read about men who have had heart attacks. But you never read about a woman having a heart attack. I think women still feel embarrassed about being sick. I'm sure some even conceal the fact they had a heart attack and survived it. Why? I don't know—perhaps they fear they'll lose

TAKE HEART

- *While depression is common after heart surgery, there are things you can do to lessen its impact on your life. Many people report that attending the hospital's cardiac rehabilitation classes boosts their spirits, since the class members offer support and encouragement. Exercise is a natural mood booster. And don't be afraid to tell your doctor how you've been feeling—if appropriate, he or she can prescribe antidepressant medications to help you through your recovery period.*

- *It often takes 4 to 6 weeks to start feeling better after heart surgery. Be patient with yourself—your body will heal, it just needs time!*

their job or they'll appear vulnerable to their friends and family. Fortunately, people are becoming more open about discussing things like this, and I hope that trend continues. I think it's especially important that women who have had cardiac problems share their experiences and the knowledge they have gained with other women, so that we can all learn from it. By being informed, we can save lives.

Today, when my son and I say our prayers together, we always ask to be kept safe and to be kept healthy. We say this because we both know that as long as you're safe and healthy, you're fine. I keep a quotation from Goethe with me now: "Be bold, and mighty forces will come to your aid." Heart patients should remember those words, because they work.

DIFFERENT SYMPTOMS, BUT THE SAME DISEASE

The number one killer of women is: _____ (hint: breast cancer isn't the answer).

It's heart disease, though you'd probably never know it from women's magazines and public service announcements. While other diseases seem to get better PR, it's heart disease that silently kills hundreds of thousands of women each year.

Part of the tragedy of this lack of PR is that many women aren't aware that the symptoms of heart disease in a woman can be very different from those in a man. This can be particularly deadly in the case of a heart attack. For example, the chest pain pattern that's experienced during a heart attack is different for women. In many cases, a woman who is having a heart attack will feel angina pain on either her left or right side, rather than in the middle of her chest, which is where a man typically feels it. In addition, women are more likely than men to experience shortness of breath during a heart attack. And women sometimes react differently than men do when given a nitroglycerin tablet during a heart attack. The tablet may act faster in a woman than it would in a man, or there are also cases where it doesn't work at all. Doctors and emergency room personnel need to be aware of these differences.

The tests used to diagnose heart disease can also have complications when used on women. For instance, EKGs are frequently falsely positive in women when they exercise, so an exercise stress test needs to be interpreted differently in the case of a woman as compared to a man. And studies like helium scans, which use radioisotopes, look positive quite frequently in women. This is because radioisotopes get reduced by the breast, which is in just the right place to produce a defect that can suggest disease.

Unfortunately, all the early studies on heart disease were done on men because doctors didn't think women were at risk for it because they had the protection of estrogen. Of course, now we know that when women's estrogen levels decline after menopause, their risk for cardiac disease escalates.

Women need to let their doctors know they want to make their heart health a priority. I recommend that all women ask their doctors for advice on what they can do to prevent heart disease. If the doctor hesitates or shrugs the problem off as irrelevant for a woman, she should find a new doctor.

—GERALD POHOST, M.D., *chief of the division of cardiovascular medicine at the University of Southern California in Los Angeles*

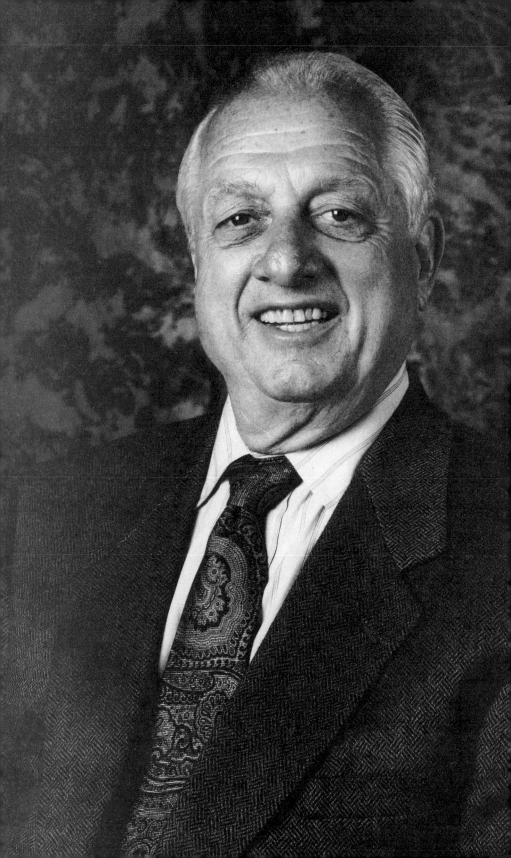

TOMMY LASORDA

Today, Tommy Lasorda's official title is Vice President of Enthusiasm for the Los Angeles Dodgers. Prior to this, he managed the team for 20 years, bringing the Dodgers a pair of World Series championships, four National League pennants, and six divisional crowns. In 1997, he was inducted into the National Baseball Hall of Fame. Two weeks later, Tommy retired from his job and that familiar #2 jersey. After he stepped down as manager, the Dodgers renamed the road outside of their Vero Beach, Florida, spring training site—what else?—Tommy Lasorda Lane.

"There are too many people walking the streets of this country who don't want to get a checkup because they are fearful of something being wrong. But knowledge is power, and regular checkups can save your life."

I was Master of Ceremonies one evening at the Cedars Sinai Sports Spectacular in 1997. We had just finished a game. Mike Piazza hit a home run in the bottom of the ninth and we won 2–1. I felt great, and we went to the affair and I said to my wife, Jo, "Is it hot in here?" She said no and I said, "Well, it sure seems warm." So we sat at the table and when it was time, I went up on the stage and did what I had to do.

The evening came to an end, and while we were driving home, all of a sudden my stomach started hurting. When we got home, Jo said she was going to call the doctor, but I told her not to, and that I'd feel better in the morning. She called him anyway and told him my stomach was bothering me, and he said to take some Mylanta. We didn't have any of that stuff in the house, so she went out and bought some and I took it.

The next day was an off day. It was a Monday and I was scheduled to speak at a black-tie hospital dinner that night. But when I called the Dodgers team physician, Dr. Michael Melman, and told him about my symptoms, he told me to get to Centinela Hospital for some tests. I did, and after the tests were finished, he told me I should stay there overnight. I said, "I'm not doing that, for Christ's sake, I gotta go. I gotta do this dinner."

He was having none of my arguments. "You want me to call Peter O'Malley (the Dodgers owner)?" he threatened. So I reluctantly agreed to stay overnight at the hospital.

He checked my stomach. And while he was doing that, I said, "You know, last night I broke out into a sweat." He looked at me and said, "Uh-oh." He brought in Dr. Anthony Reid, who is a cardiologist, and they hooked me up to machines and took an EKG and did some bloodwork. Then, after a while, Dr. Reid said, "Tommy, you've had a heart attack."

"A heart attack?" I repeated. "I had a stomachache. I give people heart attacks, I don't get 'em!"

I ended up having an angioplasty right away. The team was on the road by this time, and I figured, "Okay, I'll get through this and then go down and manage again." After it was over, Dr. Reid came back into my room and scared the hell out of me. He said, "Look, there's a 40 percent chance this is going to happen again and you're going to be back."

"40 percent?" I repeated in amazement. I didn't want to do this again.

"You've Found Your Answer"

I was released from the hospital a few days later, and by this time, everyone knew what had happened. I had phone calls

HEART ATTACK SYMPTOMS

While heart attack symptoms can vary from person to person and tend to present themselves differently in women than in men, here are the four basic signs that you might be having a heart attack. If you experience chest discomfort along with one or more of the other three symptoms, call 9-1-1 immediately.

Chest discomfort. Often described as a feeling of pressure or squeezing, the discomfort may last only a few minutes or may go away and then return. This is angina. It usually isn't as severe as "the Hollywood Heart Attack." In fact, some victims say they didn't feel any heaviness in their chest whatsoever; instead they felt as if they had eaten too much.

Pain. You might feel pain in one or both arms, or sometimes, you might even feel it in your neck and/or jaw. Many patients say they felt as though they had an upset stomach. Others felt pain in their backs.

Nausea. This common symptom may be accompanied by a sudden feeling of lightheadedness or unusual sweating.

Shortness of breath. It is difficult to breathe even when you're not active.

from everywhere and everyone, but my mind was really focused on getting back into the game. I was supposed to go in and talk to Peter O'Malley about coming back to work, and I walked up that little incline to get into the ballpark and suddenly I just felt so tired. I thought to myself, "Damn, how can I go down there and manage a ball club at 1:00 or 2:00 in the afternoon, do the game, and then do all the stuff after the game and get home at 11:00 or 12:00 when I'm so tired?"

When I finally did get to Peter's office, he of course wanted to know what my decision was going to be about coming back to work. I said, "You don't mind if Jo and I walk out of here for a minute, do you?"

He told me to go ahead. We walked outside Peter's office and I said, "What do you think?"

Jo said, "Tommy, nobody is going to be able to help you make this decision. You are the one who's going to have to say whether you want to go or not."

I said to her, "You know something? Something is telling me not to go down there."

"Well, you've found your answer," she said.

I had already talked with my cardiologist about retiring. He said that it was a decision I was going to have to make on my own, but that I needed to keep in mind the fact that I obviously see and have always seen my job as a 24-hour-a-day commitment. So even though I had only a small heart attack and my prognosis was excellent, I have a very grueling occupation and schedule. He said that to continue doing it as I have been doing it is an awful lot. I know what he was trying to tell me, but I've always been the guy to make the decisions that have to be made.

After my discussion with Jo, I went back in there and told Peter, "I just don't feel like I can go down there and do it the way I do it—you know, my way."

And you know what he told me? "Well, I'm glad you said that. And now I'm going to tell you something: You are now a vice president of this ball club." That stunned me. I never expected anything like that.

Given the fact that I had managed my team for 2 decades, it might seem surprising that I was able to make the decision to retire so quickly. But I realized I just couldn't go back down there and be myself. See, I knew that if I were the type of guy who stands in the dugout and doesn't move, like a lot of managers do, I probably could have kept going down there. But I can't do that. I'm out there screaming and hollering at the umpires or the ball players because that's my style.

And, honestly, I didn't want to end up like some of my buddies. I thought about Don Drysdale, who was announcing games for us in 1992. In July of that year, we were playing in Montreal, and after the game I went up on the elevator with him at our hotel and I said, "Let's meet for breakfast." He agreed. So that morning, I called him. He never showed up for breakfast. He never showed up at the ballpark. I told my traveling secretary, "You better check his room." They had to break the door down. He was dead—it was a heart attack. He was 55 years old.

I also thought of my own coach, Don McMahon, dying in my arms right there on the field. It was during batting practice in July of 1987. He was out pitching and I was in my office. When I came onto the field, he was lying by the dugout. I held him while we all waited for the ambulance to come. I kept telling him, "Don't die, don't die, keep holding on, Don," but he died right there. He was 57. It was a heart attack, too.

When it came time for me to face facts, I said, "Uh-uh. I want to live and see my granddaughter graduate from college. That's it; everything has to come to an end. All great things have to come to an end." And then when the doctor told me I have a 40 percent chance of it coming back, it just made my decision even easier. I think I made the right move. That was 1996. I'm 75 now.

That's not to say, though, that I didn't have to go back to the hospital. It turned out that Dr. Reid was right. About 3 months later, I was back in again. I had been walking in New York City (we weren't playing a ballgame, I was just there for some event). The pressure in my chest came out of nowhere. I could feel something inside that just wasn't right, but I didn't do anything about it until I got back home. I do remember it was a different feeling than I'd had before. I went to see Dr. Reid again, and he put me back in the hospital for another angioplasty. Since then, I've felt great, but I do worry. I'm like one of those cars that comes out of Earl Shieb—they look great on the outside, but you don't know what the hell's happening under the hood.

A Resolution to *Not* Live Like I Did Before

Before the heart attack, I used to eat everything that wasn't tied down. I ate anything, and I ate late at night. Whatever. We played in different time zones, and I started paying attention to

TAKE HEART

- *Be an active participant in your health. Schedule regular checkups with your doctor to keep an eye on your blood pressure and cholesterol levels. Being informed is one of the best defenses against heart disease.*
- *Knowing what to do in the event of a heart attack will save time and significantly improve your chances of making a full recovery. Be familiar with the warning signs, explain to your family the importance of calling 9-1-1 instead of driving to the ER in their own car, and write out a list of medications you're taking and those you're allergic to, and keep it in your wallet.*

my stomach instead of the clock. I used to eat a lot of pasta and a lot of eggs and sandwiches—I loved going to the deli or ordering hamburgers. And I used to eat all sorts of fried foods. But after my heart attack, all that changed. No more.

Yet when it comes to diet, I'll admit I'm just as guilty as everyone else is. When you get out of the hospital, you feel good and you start living life like you did before. That's what I'm trying *not* to do right now. I'm trying to lose some weight and eat properly. Before, I never worried about anything I ate. I never thought I'd have a heart attack. And I thought when you did have a heart attack, you'd get pains and all that stuff. I was wrong on both counts.

After my heart attack, I served as a spokesman for the American Heart Association. I traveled the country trying to impress upon people the need to go get a checkup. I believe you need to find out about your health status because if there is something wrong, you better get it checked out and taken care of. There are too many people walking the streets of this country who don't want to get a checkup because they are fearful of something being wrong. But knowledge is power, and regular checkups can save your life. A lot of people heard my voice. I remember a lady called me at my office. She had heard me say that sweating for no apparent reason is one warning sign of a heart attack. Her husband was having that happen, so she called an ambulance even though he kept saying, "I'm okay, it's just something I ate." Well, an hour later, he was having bypass surgery. He's alive today, I'm proud to say.

⁘⠊⠕⁘

The Doctor's Notes:
IN THE ER WITH TOMMY LASORDA

ANTHONY REID, M.D., of the Tommy Lasorda Heart Institute at Centinela Hospital in Inglewood, California

Most people think heart attacks come on strong and are unmistakable. It's true that for many people, having a heart attack feels like you have an elephant standing on your chest. But many times, it's more subtle, and I think that was the case for Tommy Lasorda. Tough guy that he is, he has a "put up with it and work through it" attitude. But certainly his symptoms of nausea, a sensation of warmth, and sweating are classic heart attack symptoms. And sometimes, that's all you get, particularly in situations that involve the right coronary artery, which was the case with Tommy.

The truth is, heart attack symptoms can vary widely. Some people have such severe symptoms that they can't move, or they lose consciousness. Unfortunately, one-third of all people having heart attacks die suddenly. But sometimes heart attacks can be less persuasive and the symptoms more subtle. Tommy thought his was an upset stomach, and you may hear that from a lot of heart patients. Nausea or upset stomach without chest pain is not an unusual or atypical presentation to me.

When Tommy came into the hospital, we did an EKG as part of the routine evaluation. The test was abnormal, and blood studies confirmed a heart attack. We also did an angiogram, which is a diagnostic study in which you put a catheter into the heart and look at the three coronary arteries. The EKG had already indicated that the problem was in one of the arteries along the interior wall. I explained to Tommy that we needed to do the angiogram to determine if there was more than just one area of blockage and also to determine the risk of additional heart attacks. We scheduled an angiogram for the next day.

Tommy was given a group of medications to limit the size of the heart attack, help preserve heart muscle, and reduce the workload on his heart. We also gave him aspirin to thin his blood. The angiogram takes about an hour to do. Tommy was awake, and one reason we like to do it this way is to show the patient what's going on. There's a monitor at the side of the table, and you can point out where the occluded vessels are. In Tommy's case, there was only one significant area—it was a small vessel, the distal aspect of the right coronary artery. There was a residual high-grade narrowing of the vessel in that spot, resulting in reduced coronary blood flow. The other two arteries were okay, and his heart muscle was in good shape. I recommended that we do an angioplasty to open the vessel. He understood and was agreeable, and we went ahead and did it at that time.

Whenever possible, our approach is to do the angioplasty right after an angiogram determines that a blockage exists. There are situations where you need to do other things; for instance, if there is a lesion in a coronary artery (a change in its structure caused by the buildup of fats or calcium), we want to treat it with medication for a period of hours before doing the angioplasty. But whenever possible, our preference is to do the angioplasty immediately. It's usually the patient's preference as well to get it all over with as quickly as possible.

We always have a surgeon standing by when we do an angioplasty because 5 percent of the time, we won't be successful. For instance, a patient getting an angioplasty might need to have coronary bypass surgery immediately. So we make the whole hospital aware and get all of our equipment ready. We did that in Tommy's case, though fortunately it was unnecessary.

I remember that as we were doing the angioplasty, Tommy asked me if his blood was blue because "he bleeds

Dodger blue." I told him, "Yes indeed, Tommy, it is blue." I didn't tell him I grew up in Cincinnati and historically, we just hated the Dodgers—because we could never beat them. They always had Koufax and Drysdale out there. It was only much later that I confessed this to him. Still, Tommy hasn't held it against me!

The second time I saw him, Tommy told me about feeling pressure in his chest while walking in New York City. I was aware he hadn't had a second heart attack, but what he did experience was a second angina episode. That was when I told him that we were going to have to do some more testing. The tests determined that his right coronary artery had once again narrowed. Tommy had been warned that this was a possibility, and now it was obvious that's what had happened. So we did a second angioplasty. Today, Tommy's doing fine. ■

ANGIOPLASTY 101

In 2000, more than one million angioplasties were performed in the United States. This procedure opens blocked arteries and allows blood to flow to the heart, saving many people from having a heart attack.

Angioplasties are performed only at hospitals that have cardiac surgery units, since in about 5 percent of cases, the procedure will be unsuccessful and cardiac surgery will be required. According to the experts at the Cleveland Clinic Heart Center, here's what you can expect if your doctor says you need an angioplasty:

- After giving you medication to relax and sedate you, the doctor numbs a site on your groin or arm with local anesthesia. Next, the doctor inserts a sheath (a thin plastic tube) into an artery (usually, this is the femoral artery in the groin, although the procedure is sometimes done through the brachial artery on the inside of the elbow). A long, narrow, hollow tube called a catheter is passed through the sheath and guided up through the blood vessel to the arteries in your heart.
- A small amount of contrast material is injected through the catheter. Using fluoroscopy (a continuous x-ray), the doctor views the blood vessels, valves, and heart chambers on a TV screen. Blockages are now visible.

◆ If necessary, your blood pressure and heartbeat will be regulated by medicine that is given through an IV in your arm. You will remain awake during the procedure, which usually takes about 1½ to 2½ hours to complete. The preparation and recovery time will add several hours.

◆ Once the blocked area of an artery is found, the physician will open it using one of four possible techniques:

Balloon angioplasty: The catheter is placed where the blockage of plaque begins and a balloon on the end of the catheter is opened, compressing the plaque against the artery wall. Blood is now able to flow through the artery once again.

Stent: In many patients, once the artery is opened by a balloon, a stent is placed to hold the artery open. It is a fine mesh tube that remains in place to provide support inside your coronary artery.

Atherectomy: Fat and plaque are shaved from the walls of the artery by a catheter with a special diamond-shaped tip. This allows blood to resume flowing through the artery.

Rotoblation: This is similar to a drill that pushes through the plaque and opens the artery.

◆ Once the catheter and the sheath are removed, either a small plug will be placed inside the hole in the artery to seal the hole, or a clamp or a heavy sandbag will be placed over the incision area for an hour to stop the bleeding. You will need to lie flat and keep the affected leg or arm straight according to your doctor's orders. A stitch or seal will be used to close the wound, or pressure will be applied for a period of time.

After leaving the hospital, you will want to keep the following considerations in mind:

- ◆ Although some bruising is normal, you should call your doctor if you have any unusual swelling, pain, or bleeding where the catheter was inserted.
- ◆ Your doctor will provide you with instructions for the care of your wound site; however, you should also be alert for signs of infection, such as increased redness, fever, warmth, or drainage at the wound site.
- ◆ After angioplasty, about 30 to 40 percent of patients will experience a repeat blockage of the arteries (this is called restenosis) in the first 6 months. That number decreases to 15 to 20 percent when a stent is implanted, and goes down even further if a medicated stent is used (this contains drugs that will keep plaque from attaching to the artery wall). It is important to call your physician if you notice a return of symptoms, such as angina or chest discomfort, excessive shortness of breath, or activity intolerance. If restenosis occurs, further intervention will be required.

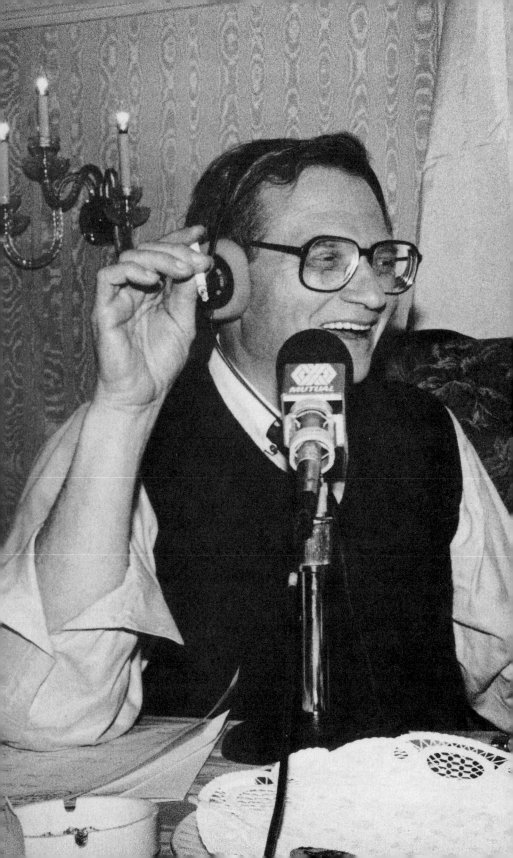

PART TWO

The Diagnosis

*"You must do the things you
think you cannot do."*
—**Eleanor Roosevelt**

My hospital stay lasted 5 days. I was given a stress test where I walked on a treadmill while hooked to monitors so that the doctors could measure my heart's response to physical exertion. It didn't take them long to decide I was in need of another angiogram. The result revealed I had one artery that was 90 percent blocked and two others that were in trouble. I was in worse shape than when I had this done just a few years earlier.

This meant we had to go to the next step: an angioplasty. A catheter would again be inserted into an artery in my groin and sent up into the area of the blockage. It doesn't remove anything; but instead, a balloon widens the artery by pushing back the obstructive plaque against the wall of the artery, thereby increasing blood flow. The procedure was done the following day.

By now, the wire services had the story that I was recuperating from a heart attack, and the hospital was getting calls and flowers and gifts from viewers and listeners all over the country.

Frank Sinatra sent a huge basket of flowers with a note that said "Anything you need. Frank." Raymond Burr sent orchids. Washington, D.C., restaurant owner Duke Zeibert brought a cheesecake—but, for obvious reasons, the hospital wouldn't allow him to bring it past the admissions desk, much less carry it to my room. My agent, Bob Woolf, flew from Boston to sit with me for a while and offer encouragement. Bob had undergone bypass surgery, and he calmly told me how heart care has become state of the art and that I'm fortunate because everyone in this hospital is the best in their respective professions. No, it didn't make me feel better at all. I was in complete shock.

Herb Cohen, my boyhood friend from Brooklyn, came directly from the airport after flying in from one of his negotiation seminars. When you face a suddenly uncertain future, it's good to spend time talking about the past. That's how a person can figure out where they stand. So we spoke about growing up along Bayshore Avenue and about people we knew from Lafayette High School. But when everyone left, I was always wide awake and found myself thinking, again, "I can't believe I've just had a heart attack. That's something that happens to someone else." The it-won't-happen-to-me logic is common and—from the perspective of experience—it's ridiculous. But that's an understanding you gain only in hindsight.

One evening after visiting hours were over, two faces appeared at the door of my room. It was Martin Sheen and homeless activist Mitch Snyder. Sheen was in town conducting research for a movie he was doing about Snyder's life. (Mitch had been a guest on my radio show whenever the news of the day had to do with the national trend of increased homelessness in cities. He was a constant pain to any member of Congress trying to cut federal funds for homeless shelters.) The three of us shot the breeze about all sorts of things, and it felt good to get off the subject of hearts for a while. But then Sheen told me about the heart attack he had at age 36 while filming *Apocalypse Now* in the Philippines. He had even been given last rites. Suddenly, I didn't feel so alone. Before he and Mitch left, Sheen pulled a crystal from his pocket and put it in my hand. He told me it had energy and that it brought luck. After we said goodbye, I held the clear quartz rock in my hand for the rest of the night. If you want the truth, I didn't feel any energy, but it sure felt good to have something, other than thoughts, to hang on to. I still have it.

When I was released from the hospital, Tammy picked me up and gave me a ride back to my condo overlooking the Potomac River and the Washington, D.C., waterfront. On the way, I reached into my pocket and found the opened pack of cigarettes that I had taken with me 6 days earlier. I rolled down the window and tossed them out onto the pavement. I know, it is littering and I'd have gladly paid the $200 fine had we been pulled over. My smoking days had come to an end. Since then, I haven't had a desire to light up—not after dinner, not after sex, not while reading, and certainly not while being driven to the hospital! Some people get hypnotized, others go to classes after work, but me? I have a heart attack to quit smoking. There were no withdrawal symptoms, but going through a heart attack isn't my recommendation for a way to stop.

Bob Woolf had arranged for me to go to Miami and take in

some baseball games. Spring training was in full swing, and I was eager to see uniforms other than the ones belonging to doctors and nurses. On the plane to Miami, I was sitting with 1968 presidential candidate Eugene McCarthy and former Secretary of State Al Haig (yes, it was a bipartisan effort). A passenger got on the plane, saw the three of us, and said, "Damn, if this plane goes down, I'm not going to be in the first paragraph." Haig leaned over and told me he had read about my heart attack and mentioned that I may be a candidate for bypass surgery. He had had the procedure and was quick to say it was a piece of cake. I didn't pay a lot of attention because bypass surgery was something that always happened to someone else (yeah, I know what you're thinking). I was more focused on two things when I got to Florida: (1) Will the Baltimore Orioles improve their pitching and (2) Where is the closest hospital to the Fountainbleau, where I was staying?

For months after leaving the hospital, I slept with the lights on, and I always knew how far away I was from an emergency room—no matter what city I was in. Miami was the perfect place to regroup after what I had just been through, and although it was clear the Orioles weren't going to do very well in the upcoming season, I came home ready to jump into work. In fact, my first radio show had cardiologists Dr. Levy and Dr. Katz as guests, and we spent a few hours talking about heart attacks. In retrospect, I think the show was medicinal for me because with all the telephone lines blinking and all the questions coming in for the doctors, I suddenly understood that this is something that is happening to a lot of people, and that lifestyle is a big reason. If you set aside having genes that are prone to heart disease, you realize that you really do have a good degree of control over it.

I changed from eating stuff like breaded veal chops, steaks, and fettuccini alfredo to salads with turkey and tuna. I started walking. And probably best of all, I didn't start lecturing others about how to live their lives. Anonymous had it right: "If it is to be, it's up to me."

But one morning in late summer during my morning walk along the Key Bridge, which crosses the Potomac from Virginia into Georgetown, I realized I was short of breath. It was one of Washington D.C.'s "triple-H" days—hazy, hot, and humid. I wrote it off as nothing more than that, along with the fact that I may have been breathing in the fumes of all the cars that were stuck in one of Georgetown's famous traffic jams. Yeah, there is always a reason for why something can't be what it is. The shortness of breath started happening more frequently (a few days later, it really hit me while I was walking through the San Francisco airport, where there is no hazy-hot-and-humid any-where), so I decided it was time to pay a visit to Dr. Katz again.

I did a stress test while hooked to an EKG machine at the hospital where I had spent 6 nights a few months earlier. After 90 seconds, Dr. Katz said, "Okay, Mr. King, that's enough." I thought to myself, "Gee, these machines are getting faster at giving results." We walked across the street to his office, and that's when I heard a word he hadn't used since that February morning when we first met: "concern." Dr. Katz told me he was "concerned because the stress test was positive," which I thought to be a good thing. It wasn't. He told me it was obvious the blockage had returned and that I was now a prime candidate for bypass surgery. My medical records were sent to Dr. Blumenthal in New York for a second opinion, and within a few weeks, he called and said he concurred with Dr. Katz.

I told Dr. Blumenthal that I was going to be in contract negotiations with CNN, I had a book tour coming up, my career was starting to really fly, and I had already booked speaking engagements around the country for a lot of money and . . .

"Larry," he interrupted me, "you have to get this surgery done and it doesn't have to be done tomorrow—but that doesn't mean it can wait until next summer either."

Like that moment in the emergency room when I was told I had just had a heart attack, I realized, again, that the way things are, and the way I think things are, are different—very different. It was now time to stop with the excuses and, once again, face the music—even though I didn't like the tune I was hearing.

"Who should I have do this?" I asked.

Dr. Blumenthal didn't miss a beat. "Dr. Wayne Isom," he said. "That's who I'd have operate on my father." With a recommendation like that, I'd found my answer.

Within a few weeks, the date of December 1 had been set. I was terrified. And during this time, I kept having one recurring thought: Maybe, I reasoned, they'll find a cure before I go in. Look, sometimes a guy just grabs at whatever he can hang on to.

On the day before I went to New York for "the grand opening," as everyone started calling it, I had to be at the radio studio to record some commentaries that would run while I was recuperating, and I remember walking with my radio producer to grab a quick lunch. I stopped in front of a pizza place and looked at the double cheese offerings.

"Larry," he cautioned, "you can't do that."

"What are they gonna do?" I argued. "What does it matter at this point?" We both had a lunch of cheese pizza that day.

That night, Bill Cosby was on my television show and Art Buchwald was a guest on my radio show. In both interviews, I was there, but I wasn't there. The questions were automatic, and I think it was because I was listening more to my fears than I was to the conversations. Art told me he had bypass surgery and nobody made much of a big deal about it. "But Larry King," he said, having fun with me, "Larry tells everybody. This is big news. If you have a double bypass, nobody will care. If you have a triple bypass, friends will listen for 3 minutes but no longer. If you have a quadruple bypass, business acquaintances will put up with it for, maybe, 2 minutes tops. You really gotta have a quintuple bypass to get anybody to pay attention." He said it was no big deal and he'd see me for dinner when I had recuperated.

I must have heard that phrase—"it's no big deal"—793 times, and in every case, I had an answer: They are going to cut open my chest, hook my most essential blood vessels up to a machine, stop my heart, take a vein from my leg and put it in my heart, start up my heart (I hope), turn off the machine, and close me up. Let me tell you something: This is "a big deal."

Jon Miller, who at the time was the voice of the Baltimore Orioles (he's now seen on ESPN baseball coverage), had offered to drive me to Manhattan. We spent the 4 hours on the road talking about possible trades for every team in the American League before discussing trades in the National League. I just didn't want to talk about the heart anymore. It was cold and rainy outside, and inside, I was feeling the same way. Jon dropped me off at New York Hospital, and I was taken to a corner room on the 18th floor with a view of the East River. I remember the hospital's public affairs person telling me this was the same room used by the Shah of Iran when he was treated for heart disease. As she left, I turned to ask one more question, but suddenly it became clear I was the only one in the room. "The Shah of Iran?" I said to nobody. "Isn't he dead?"

Just then Bob Woolf came in and we spent a few moments talking about what I would be doing when I got out of there. He said, "Larry, 6 days from now you'll be mad as hell about some baseball team making a bad trade." I didn't believe a word he told me.

That evening, a guy walked in wearing a cowboy hat, blue jeans, and boots. "Larry King?" he asked. I looked at him from my hospital bed and figured this was someone with a mother who wanted an autograph (it's always the mother who wants an autograph). "Yes," I said.

A huge hand was extended. "Wayne Isom. You gonna do right fine, Mr. King!" I had been told Dr. Isom was one of the best bypass surgeons in the country and had great respect from cardiologists around the world. But I had pictured him as bald, with no sense of humor, wearing a white shirt and dark suit every day with the tie always tight around his neck. I wanted Dr. Wayne Isom to be a guy who always read *Heart Bypass*

Digest before breakfast and who had never been to a Yankees game. Let's just say the fellow standing at the foot of my bed wasn't what I had envisioned. He wasn't aloof. He had a Texas drawl and was smiling. I kept thinking to myself, "Oh boy, what do I do now?"

Dr. Isom pulled up a chair and went through what the next few days were going to entail. I was going to have an angiogram the next morning. That evening, I'd be given a tranquilizer. On the day of the surgery, I'd be taken to the OR early in the morning, and I'd wake up later that evening with a tube in my mouth. As for right now, he suggested I have a dinner of lamb chops or a filet mignon and fruit salad because it would be my last good meal. All I heard was "last meal." I was still terrified and remained so all the way to the operating room on Tuesday morning. To make me sleep, I was given something after my "last meal." (I had the fillet. Delicious, but if truth be told, it could have just as easily been corn flakes. Terror takes over the taste buds, too.) Whatever was in that pill worked, but I don't think I woke any more rested. The mind has a mind of its own. But when I did open my eyes that morning, it wasn't the result of bad dreams or terror. It was a nurse's calm voice and the words, "Good morning, Mr. King."

I was shaved that morning—they shave everything—and I remember just kind of lying there as if on cruise control. I wasn't thinking about anything. I knew what was going to happen in a few hours, and I was totally accepting of the fact that, damn it, they hadn't found a cure during the night. Now, to use the words of Bob Fosse in his 1987 movie *All That Jazz*, it was "showtime." I'm glad I wasn't thinking clearly enough to realize that the film is based on Fosse working too hard, smoking, drinking too much, and having a heart attack.

The last thing I remember doing before I went into the OR was answering a question: "Who is your doctor?" With a clear mind and what I thought to be a clear voice, I said "Isom." This is done to make sure the hospital has the right patient for the right procedure, even though there is a wrist band and a chart indicating the surgery to be done. After I answered the question, I was out.

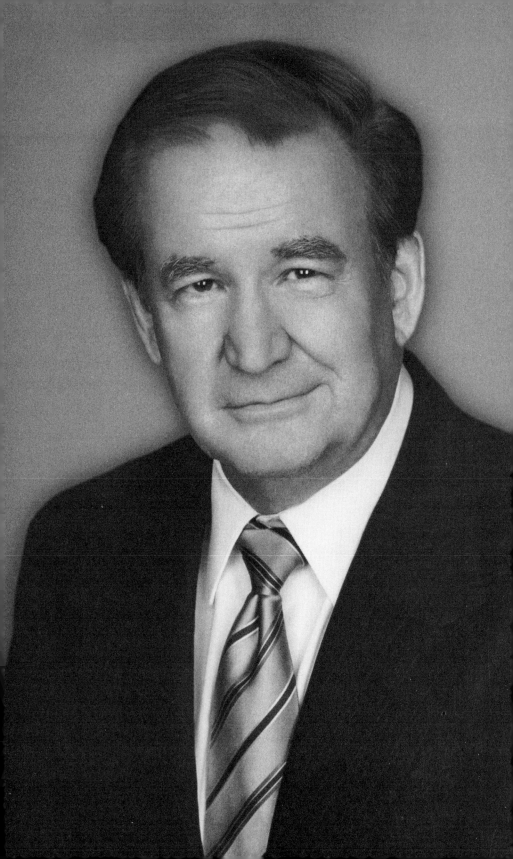

PAT BUCHANAN

Pat used to co-host a radio talk show every evening with Tom Braden that was the basis for the CNN show Crossfire—*and he has argued the "right" side of issues every night on CNN for almost 17 years. Besides being a nationally syndicated newspaper columnist, a senior advisor to three presidents (Nixon, Ford, and Reagan), an author of seven books about public policy, and a three-time presidential candidate, Pat has always been at home in a debate. He feels the words. In 1991, however, he started feeling something else—a deteriorating heart. And for once in his life, there was no debate to be held: He was going to get it fixed.*

"Get the surgery done and get it over with, and then get out and start walking right away. Have a positive attitude, and soon enough, you are going to get stronger."

When I was 42 years old, I was told during a routine physical exam that I had a heart murmur. I wasn't feeling tired or anything like that, but I definitely had a leaking aortic heart valve. So I was monitored at the Washington Hospital Center, where they used an echocardiogram machine to show the simulcast of the blood flow in and out of my heart in color.

As my physician, Dr. Maurice Sislen, and I watched all of this happening on a monitor, he would point to where blood was actually flowing back into my heart because of the defective heart valve. I remember lying there quietly listening to the rolling surf of the blood moving in and out of my heart and reflecting upon my mortality. As I listened to the "whoosh" sound my blood made, Dr. Sislen explained that I had about 5 years before I needed to have the valve replaced.

Despite what Dr. Sislen told me that day, I was able to wait 10 years before getting the surgery. Scheduling it became a problem because by the fall of 1991, I had already decided to run against President George H. W. Bush, but this was the same time the doctors were warning me that I had only a year left before the operation was no longer optional. I announced that I'd be running against Bush, and we did very well in New Hampshire. But I knew surgery was necessary.

I was starting to have symptoms that were bothering me. In 1991, during a PBS interview on *American Interests*, I had a sudden searing, cutting sensation straight down the center of my chest. It lasted for most of the show. At first I thought it was a heart attack, but because the debate was sharp and intense and the pain eventually passed, I decided it must have come from natural adrenaline. Then it happened again during an interview on *Nightline*. I thought it was just from getting nervous. But then I thought, "Wait a second, I've been doing debates for a long time. What is going on here? Am I getting old? Can't I handle it anymore?" I was also having a tough time sleeping on my left side, and my heart was pounding so hard that I could feel the thumping. I couldn't get comfortable. And this was very tough in New Hampshire because we had a campaign going. Still, I went out running almost every day and returned feeling refreshed, relaxed, and awake.

On April 15th—after the New Hampshire and Georgia primaries—I asked Dr. Sislen if I could go without surgery until after the California primary, which was June 2nd. I wanted to wait until after California because I had promised to be out there, and he said, "Yes, but . . . you can't go through November without the surgery."

At every stop from April on, the press would ask me, "Why are you staying in?" I knew I wasn't going to beat George Bush, but I had made that promise to go to California and I was going to keep it. Looking back, though, the need for heart valve surgery was taking its toll. When I went to the *Washington Times* to talk with the editorial board, a reporter wrote that all the fight had gone out of me. I would jog every day, but I was cutting off campaign events in the evening. Instead, I would have dinner and go to bed.

I didn't tell anyone I had a heart problem. I figured I'd cross that bridge when I came to it (like if and when I got the nomination). Nobody asked me about it. But if somebody had come up to me and said, "Look, I've got a report you may have to have heart surgery in the next year, is that right?" I'd have said, "Yes, that's right." But people did come up to me and ask, "How's your health?" I'd say, "Well, I run 2 miles a day" and stuff like that. Nobody paid much attention to me because nobody thought I was going to win. Once we decided on a date for the surgery, the campaign continued, but when I was back in Washington, D.C., I would go to the Washington Hospital Center and donate blood for my upcoming surgery.

The Secret Service knew what I had to do, and they'd take me over to the hospital with a police escort every time. I'd have blood taken, and it would be put in the blood bank for me under the name "John Doe" (if truth be told, I had offered to use the name Schuyler Colfax, the founder of the Republican Party, but the nurse in charge said John Doe was fine). I was worried that someone would find my name on several blood bank units and tip the press. But they'd slip me in there, I would give a unit, talk with the nurses, eat some cookies and down some juice to restore my energy, and go home. The nurses were all pledged to secrecy. I was down to 160 pounds by this time, and there are pictures that were taken of me where I looked like I was 70 years old when I was just 52.

I went out to California and campaigned, and on the Tuesday of the primary I flew to New Hampshire to say good-bye to everyone who had helped me do so well before I ended the campaign. (Despite many saying we had no chance in New Hampshire, I came in a close second to George Bush with 37 percent of the GOP vote to his 51 percent.)

FROM THE CAMPAIGN TRAIL TO A HOSPITAL ROOM

With the campaign over, I was finally able to focus on my health. I approached surgery this way: A lot of things are out of your hands, but you still need to ask questions. I called my brother, Buck, who is a doctor, and said, "Look, Shelley wants me to go to Houston or Birmingham or Cleveland for the surgery evaluation. What's your advice? My doctor says the best place to have it done is right here in Washington, D.C., in Washington Hospital Center."

My brother said, "You've got two places in D.C. that are famous—The Hospital Center and Fairfax Hospital. It's like an all-star game in making the choice between the two. Do you want to bring in DiMaggio or Williams to do your pinch-hitting for you?" His advice, coupled with the fact that this is my home and I'm comfortable here, sealed my decision to have the surgery done in Washington. This is where I grew up. I used to pass by here when I would hitchhike to school. So I went with it.

I went into the hospital on a Wednesday night. On Thursday, they did all these tests, and doctors and nurses came in to brief

BLOOD DONATIONS AND CELL SALVAGE

Patients having bypass or heart valve surgery are often in need of a transfusion to replace blood that is lost during these operations. For a number of years, patients have either received donor blood from a national blood supply or have donated their own blood (a process known as preoperative autologous donation) prior to the surgery. Donated blood has a shelf life of no more than 42 days. After this period of time, the red blood cells begin to break down, making the blood unusable.

There are some distinct benefits to donating your own blood prior to surgery. For example, some patients are hesitant to accept blood from other donors fearing it could be contaminated with hepatitis B, hepatitis C, or even HIV, despite the fact that U.S. blood suppliers take every precaution to ensure its safety. In addition, your own stored blood matches perfectly.

There is now a strong movement toward cell salvage, which uses a patient's blood that would otherwise be lost during surgery. With this technique, blood is suctioned from the incision during the operation and then filtered and centrifuged to separate the red blood cells from contaminants such as clots,

me on their roles and on what to expect. They left booklets to read and a video to watch, but I decided I didn't need to know everything. They're good at this, and they know what they're doing. Look, I don't need to read about what the mechanic is going to do to my automobile as long as he makes it go again.

tissue, and other blood products. The blood is then washed with a saline solution and returned to the patient within a few minutes. Generally, preoperative donation is not needed when cell salvage is used because the capability of cell salvage is well beyond that of donating one or two units for oneself.

Patients using their own blood are monitored for their respective red blood cell concentrations prior to surgery to ensure that their red blood cell count is adequate. The blood of an adult male is normally 42 to 54 percent red blood cells, while that of an adult woman is 38 to 44 percent. A man is considered anemic when his red blood cell count is less than 39 percent; a woman is considered anemic when her count is less than 36 percent. When patients are anemic prior to surgery, it places them at increased risk of needing a blood transfusion and makes the cell salvage process less effective. For this reason, anemic patients should have the cause of their anemia evaluated and treated prior to elective surgery.

—JONATHAN WATERS, M.D., *director of autotransfusion services at the Cleveland Clinic Foundation*

Dr. Jorge Garcia was recommended as the guy to do the job. Dr. Garcia had done heart surgery on John Whittaker, who worked with me in the Nixon White House and later became Undersecretary of the Interior. President Nixon knew Dr. Garcia as well, and I'm sure I talked to Nixon about it afterwards. So

Dr. Garcia came in and said, "Let me tell you about the surgery. Ninety-seven percent of patients live a normal life coming out of this." Being my usual self, I was going to ask, "Well, what about the other 3 percent? What do they do?" But I refrained.

I was taken down for an angiogram, a procedure where a wire is inserted into a major artery in the groin area, then run up through all the arteries in the heart to see if any are clogged and have to be bypassed. Dr. Garcia explained the need to do the angiogram this way: "If we're going to make the trip in, we might as well do the job right." Fortunately, the arteries were clean and clear. To a layman, an angiogram sounds like a dreadful and painful procedure. But while no picnic, it is relatively painless. I will tell you that the relief I felt about my arteries being clear exceeded any discomfort I experienced during that 45-minute procedure.

Thursday night before the surgery, I got a call from Vice President Dan Quayle, who said he planned a corker of a speech in Indianapolis on family values for the following Monday. I was also visited by a Filipino priest, a charismatic Catholic, who brought me Holy Communion.

Finally, I was alone. I had thought about this moment all along. The surgery was hanging over me, and I knew it was getting closer. I said, "Okay, I'm going to have to have this done. It's going to take a big block of my life and time, and it's going to be a bad hit, and it's going to take a long time to recuperate, but it has to be done." My attitude was very positive. I'm pessimistic about the world, but I'm optimistic about myself. Western civilization is going to hell in a handbasket, but I'm doing just fine. You go in there and you say to yourself, "97 percent are going to be okay, and I'm one of those guys who will come out of this just fine."

The next morning, they wheeled me down for the surgery, and while I was still lying on the gurney, they wheeled in another guy, who recognized me. We're both lying there alone, and I looked over and said, "I think I'm going ahead of you." He laughed.

I got the St. Jude valve, which is a mechanical valve. Unlike pig valves, it lasts forever; but it does mean that I have to take a blood thinner for the rest of my life.

The next thing I knew, I woke up with the mask on. I could hear voices. My wife Shelley, and my sister Bay. My overriding sensation was that I was on the verge of choking to death. As I tried to breathe, I realized that something was in my throat— the tube of the breathing machine. My mind said, "Relax, leave it alone, it's helping you breathe," but my instinct said to grab that thing and pull it out of my throat or I'd suffocate. The best I could do was squeeze Shelley's hand to let her know I could hear. Tubes were running out of my throat, nose, ankle, arm, wrist, and stomach and, of course, there was the one running up into my bladder. I felt truly awful.

All day I lay there falling asleep, awakening, and falling asleep again. Nurses kept looking in to ask if I needed another hit of morphine. The answer was always "yes." At midnight, a team came in and told me they were going to pull the breathing tube out. "Okay," I nodded. This was the single worst moment. The fluid buildup in my lungs was enormous, and as they pulled the tube out, I felt as though my insides were flowing up through my throat and were going to choke me to death before it all poured out onto my face. The expulsion of all that fluid, forced out of my now-wired chest and rib cage, was truly painful.

Early Saturday morning, they wheeled me out of the recovery area and into post-operative intensive care. I spent that day lying in pain, sleeping and, for a brief moment, reading. The *Washington Post* had a story about my operation being successful, and I was glad I hadn't tried to learn what would be done from the reading materials and video I had been given prior to surgery. The newspaper story went into detail about how my heart was stopped, I was put on a machine, and the defective valve was replaced in a procedure that took 4 hours. No thanks.

The next day I had to sit up every 2 hours and blow into a contraption that registered lung power. This was a problem because, despite my efforts, I wasn't registering well. The doctors found fluid congealing and compacting at the base of my lungs, and they were concerned about pneumonia. So they sent in a nurse specialist who beat my back with her open palms, near my kidneys, to break the fluid up. Sugar Ray Leonard couldn't have done a better job. After a second beating, I decided to start blowing into the contraption constantly until I registered satisfactorily. And when I did, the pounding was stopped.

On Track for Recovery

Each day, as more of the tubes were removed, I started to feel as though I could function again on my own. Calls and cards poured in: President and Mrs. Bush, President Reagan, President Nixon. There were enough bouquets and flower arrangements to satisfy the Corleones at the wake of the Godfather. I even had a nice note from Newt Gingrich, who had trashed me during the campaign because I was supporting a candidate running against him in the Georgia Primary (Herman Clark).

Soon I was able to walk to a cardiac rehabilitation class to which all the cardiac patients were invited after their operations. It was just down the hallway from my room, and I took a seat in the middle of a small semi-circle of a dozen or so patients. A woman with a French accent came in, showed a film, and then began to instruct us on how, henceforth, we had to conduct our lives.

She informed us that walking was essential. We were to start with long, slow walks and then with each passing day, go for longer distances. Smoking was forbidden. She began listing the foods we could eat as well as the foods we could no longer eat. After listening for 10 minutes or so about diet, I raised my hand and asked, "I haven't had bypass surgery. I had a heart valve replaced. Do I need to be in here?" The answer was no, so I excused myself. It was a brief, but moving, session. People who didn't know each other spoke prosaically about matters of life and death and about what was important to them. (A man who was a roofer was in for his second bypass and wanted to enjoy more time with his grandchildren once he was released.)

When I went home, I spent afternoons sleeping. I'd get up, do something, and then fall asleep after a few hours. This went on for weeks. It was a routine, and though I was aware that I was sleeping a lot, I viewed it as a necessary routine. Each day I felt stronger, but I also knew that I was still recovering. It took a while—longer than I had figured—but that was just fine. I think it's important for anyone going through this to be patient and not try to rush back to work and a full schedule.

Two months and 2 weeks after my surgery, I took President Bush up on his offer to let me use his family's Houston country club. (The 1992 Republican Convention was in Houston, and I had been asked to give a speech supporting the nominee and the platform on the first night.) The club had a one-mile track inside the grounds, and I would go there every day with my guys who worked with me during the campaign. I couldn't even run a mile, though. I'd walk and run, and it wasn't until the 6th day we were there when I was finally able to run a mile. I remember I came out of the shower after that run and Bush's son Neal was there, and I said, "Hi Neal, how are you doing?" He just looked at the scar running from my collarbone down my front. It's a zipper-like thing, and I could see the shock on his face.

A Changed Perspective

Based on my experience, I would advise other people to exercise and try to get themselves in the best condition they can prior to the operation because it is going to be a big hit. So give yourself a head start by trying to go in there in as good a shape as you can be. (Looking back, I probably shouldn't have waited until June. By then, I was drawn and down to 160 pounds. I probably should have had it done in the fall.)

I'd also recommend getting the operation as soon as you start to feel the symptoms—the inability to sleep, the discomfort, the pains. Get the surgery done and get it over with, and then

TAKE HEART

- *Don't put off having heart surgery. You will recover more quickly if you're strong going into the operation. And getting the surgery behind you allows you to focus on making changes in your lifestyle that will give you an even healthier future.*
- *Too busy to exercise? Try focusing on simply increasing the number of steps you take each day. For example, instead of searching for the closest parking spot, park farther away and log a few extra steps. Use the stairs instead of the elevator. And if you work in an office, walk to your co-workers' offices for one-on-one conversations instead of sending them e-mails.*

get out and start walking right away. Have a positive attitude, and soon enough, you are going to get stronger.

Still, there will be relapses in terms of strength and energy. I will tell you there are times when you think you're doing well and then you drop back. I found I would get weepy. I was stunned by that. I've always had the Irish problem where I cry at the end of movies, but it is far worse after surgery. I think it is some psychosomatic effect that happens. You are moved by feelings and stories and you feel emotional about things where before you were tougher. In this case, it's not that you start to cry, it's more a sense of emotion. You get choked up about things that you wouldn't have thought twice about prior to the surgery.

Apart from the surgery, I'm getting older, and I think that's changed my attitude. I think about just writing books and reading. The campaigns are over, and I'm not going to run again. I don't have the same ambition and drive that I used to have. I think as you get older, there are a lot of issues you really don't care about that much anymore. I've seen this on these TV shows I do. I laugh a lot more, and I don't take the partisanship as seriously.

Prior to the surgery, perhaps I was a better editorial writer and commentator than I am now in terms of passion and engagement. I was more interested in the larger issues then. But after going through something like I did, I think it's only natural that my priorities have shifted. It takes more to get me agitated and upset now. Still, my heart surgery took place the same week that North Carolina Republican Senator Jesse Helms had bypass surgery and the same week that the Reverend Donald Wildman of the Family Resource Center had cardiac surgery. So I called Helms while he was at home recovering and said, "Don't tell me there isn't a conspiracy. . . ."

THE DOCTOR'S NOTES:
HEART VALVE REPLACEMENT

MAURICE SISLEN, M.D., associate clinical professor
in the department of medicine at the
George Washington University Medical Center in Washington, D.C.

There came a point when Pat Buchanan's left ventricle could not compensate adequately for the blood it actually had to pump twice. Because of a faulty valve, some of the blood that had been pumped out of his heart would leak back in, meaning that it had to be pumped out again. This made extra work for the muscle, which then made it less efficient.

While there have been several changes in the design of replacement valves, doctors are essentially using the same kind of valves and doing basically the same procedures now that we used when Pat had his surgery. I'll tell you, the state of the art was pretty well advanced by the time Pat got his valve. He was given a mechanical valve rather than a pig valve because of his long life expectancy. A pig valve is used only for older people, and patients who have them don't require any anticoagulation medication.

Pat's mechanical valve functions similarly to the way his original valve did when it was working correctly, except that it is more prone to infection than a normal valve. In addition, because these valves are mechanical and will show some wear and tear from time to time, they are not guaranteed; patients may need to have them replaced. Pat is on anticoagulant therapy, and he has to take antibiotics because he is prone to complications from any bacteria that are floating around in his bloodstream from things like dental procedures. In most individuals, the bacteria are of no consequence, but in patients with a mechanical valve, bacteria can land on the valve and cause an infection because there's no resistance to the bacteria. Therefore Pat, and others like him, must take an antibiotic an hour or so before any dental procedure. Still, this is a relatively minor inconvenience given the high quality of life enjoyed by most patients with replacement heart valves. ■

Four Things to Know About "The Tube"

While many patients dread the breathing tube that is used during and immediately after cardiac surgery, being educated about what to expect can go a long way in reducing this fear and anxiety. The endotracheal tube attaches the patient to a ventilator, which breathes for him or her during cardiac surgery and in the ICU. It is placed into the trachea (the windpipe) leading to the lungs once the patient is put under anesthesia prior to the procedure. The tube is approximately 1 foot long and measures 8 to 9 millimeters in diameter for adult men, and 7 to 8 millimeters for adult women. (Occasionally, a smaller tube may be used for actors, actresses, or other people who are dependent on their voice. However, breathing with a smaller tube can be more difficult than with a tube of normal size because the rate that oxygen-containing gas is taken in is decreased.)

I make four points with my patients when I discuss what to expect with the tube during surgery and its use in the ICU:

1. *Don't be scared of it.* When you wake up after surgery, you aren't going to be able to talk. There will be a sense that a lot is going on around you, but it shouldn't be construed in any way that there is a problem. You will wake up on your own. The chemical agents that were administered through an IV in your arm to put you to sleep are relatively predictable, meaning they will last for a certain

amount of time (usually no longer than 4 to 6 hours after leaving the operating room).

2. *Don't fight the ventilator.* Yes, it is disconcerting to try to breathe this way. Some people describe the experience as breathing through a straw; they feel as though they can't take a deep breath, when in fact they are breathing just as deeply as normal. Further, because your chest has been opened, deep breaths may be painful.

3. *Be prepared for more than one tube.* In some instances, you may also have a nasogastric tube (a tube that is placed in the nose and runs into the stomach). This tube clears the stomach of fluid and air that builds up during the operation and prevents the stomach from developing a buildup of gas while you're on the ventilator. Or, instead of a nasogastric tube, your doctor might choose to insert an orogastric tube (a tube that runs from the mouth to the esophagus and into the stomach).

4. *Try to remember that you likely won't need the breathing tube for very long.* The tube is usually removed within a few hours of coming into the ICU after surgery. Once doctors are confident your blood pressure and heart rate are stable, and your lung function is normal, the tube is removed. You will be able to talk, but will be given an oxygen mask to ease your transition to breathing room air.

—JOHN R. COOPER, JR., M.D., *associate chief of cardiovascular anesthesiology at Texas Heart Institute at St. Luke's Episcopal Hospital, Texas Medical Center, in Houston*

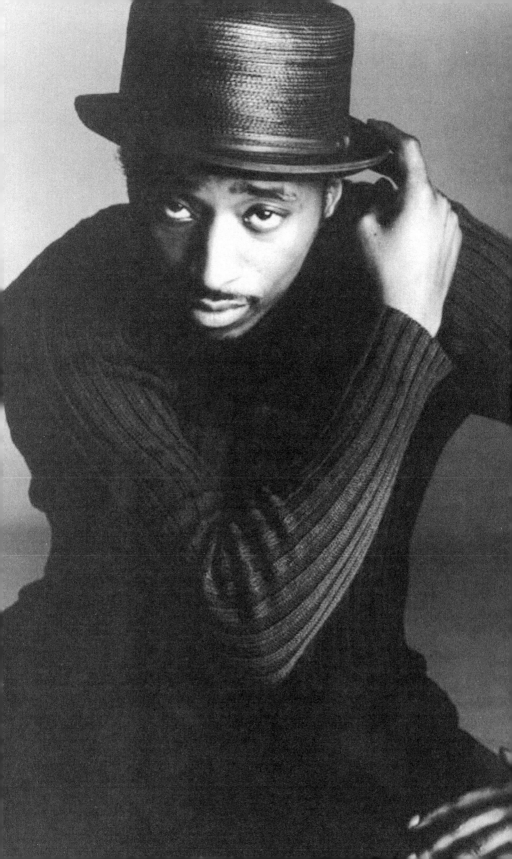

EDDIE GRIFFIN

*Eddie made a name for himself doing
standup comedy before making a number
of popular movies including* DysFunktional
Family, Undercover Brother, *and* Scary
Movie 3. *He also played Sammy Davis Jr.
in a remake of that singer and "rat pack"
member's life story. But it was while doing a
UPN TV show called* Malcolm and Eddie *in
1996 that he learned his heart was in
trouble.*

"If you make up your mind to do something— whether it's improving your health or choosing a career—you have to stick with it. Yes, it's hard to do, but it really is mind over matter. You determine what happens in your life."

The day I had my heart attack started like any other. I got up that morning as usual, felt energetic, and headed out to the studio, where we were working on an episode of *Malcolm and Eddie*. We worked all day, until finally it was something like "take 16" of a scene where I had to dance a salsa number. It was late afternoon, sometime after 5:00 P.M., and we were going to tape the show that evening. But doing this scene was taking a long time because we had the only Latino woman in California who can't salsa. (I still don't know who did that casting.) And that was when I started to feel a little tingling on my left side, but I didn't pay any attention to it. I was finding it a little rough to breathe, and then they called a time-out for dinner.

I went upstairs to my dressing room, ate a couple pieces of beef, and realized my tongue was feeling real acidy. I spit out the beef and thought to myself, "Maybe they're right and beef ain't good for you." I still wasn't getting it that I was having a heart attack, and I sat there trying to eat something for 5 minutes.

Suddenly I felt everything lock up on my left side, and my tongue felt like it was hanging out, and I was trying to get my breath. One of my friends looked at me and said, "Man, you don't look too good." He said he was going to get the paramedics. I remember telling him, "You might want to *run* out and get the paramedics." They always had a team of medical people on the set—and I'm glad they did. They gave me a nitroglycerin tablet and told me to keep it under my tongue, and it helped me breathe better. That worked quick. Then I was put on a stretcher and put in the ambulance. I remember seeing this screen above me and it was blipping, and all of a sudden it went blank. I thought, "Okay, I guess I'm dead."

But I always felt like I was going to come through this okay. I think you know when it's time to go permanently. I always felt I was going to be all right. I could feel the ambulance turn a corner, and the next thing I knew I was hit with the jumper cables. We pulled up to what I later learned was Brotman Medical Center in Culver City.

I do recall hearing the words "heart attack" from a doctor at the hospital. As he said it, I was thinking, "I pretty much figured that part out. I'm the one who's being attacked here. It didn't take a rocket scientist for you to come here with your white lab coat to figure all of that out!"

The doctors decided I needed to have angioplasty because a major artery was clogged. While they did this, I kept saying to myself, "No more bacon sandwiches." I did tell the medical team working on me, "Look, I've been dead once today, so if you mess up, that's okay, we'll just be dead together." They kind of got a kick out of that. I was making jokes. I think you just have to be a fighter to the end. If you roll over and play dead, you are going to die. But if you fight and try to stay positive, I believe it can make a difference. You can help determine the outcome.

Later, the doctor told me that stress causes the liver to deliver maximum amounts of cholesterol. I believe to this day that the stress of doing *Malcolm and Eddie* almost killed me. I was arguing with the network. I was arguing with writers who I thought weren't funny and this, that, and the other. I believed that what they wanted me to do didn't make any sense. I come from the stand-up world, and I know what's funny. I tried out stuff every night myself, and then I would try out a script and see plain as day it wasn't funny—and, well, that's stress. And then it became clear that all I was really doing was selling soap and soda pop. After a while, I could see I was what comes on between the commercials. It's that old saying, "Money ain't everything." I knew that all too well sitting in that hospital.

On top of the stress of the show, I was eating a bad diet. Let me tell you, soul food is nothing but grease. You get corn bread and you gotta have butter on it. You get blackeyed peas and you get fatback in it. Fried chicken is always greasy. Pork chops are always greasy. Plus, I was smoking like a chimney—at least two packs a day. I was a young man, so I was in the stage where I thought I was invincible. My heart attack changed that tune real fast.

The Center of the Storm

My parents were on the set the day I had the heart attack, so I spent most of my time in the hospital, it seems, trying to calm my mother down. I think it's probably worse for the family than it is for the guy in the center of the storm. That's where it's calm, but all around it's the family and friends who are panicking. But when things quieted down and I was left alone, all I could think about was, "How do I get out of this hospital?" In fact, I got out of bed and figured, "Okay, you fixed my heart, let me test it. I don't want to get out of here and get into a basketball game and be right back in here." So I wandered the halls—even tried some jogging. I did my own test. I did well, and I guess that means the doctors did well, too.

I didn't hear from anybody on the set. I figured the producers were already on the phone looking for other comedians. But the thing that was the most helpful was my brother saying to me, "I'll break you out of here in the morning." I really have a thing about hospitals. I hate the smell, and I hate the look, and I couldn't wait to get out of there.

Comedy in a place like that is always better than the weeping "gee-you're-not going-to-die-are-you?" stuff. "Let me sing you a sad song." No thanks. I think it's helpful if people just come in and have a sense of humor. They ought to walk in and say, "Oh, you ain't dead yet? Well, I'll wait outside then. But since you ain't dead, you want to get up and clean this room a little bit? Make yourself useful while you're still alive, okay?"

When I came back to work, I had a sense nobody really believed I had a heart attack. Instead, they were thinking, "That Black guy must have been a crack addict." I say this because I got asked that very question a number of times by interviewers when I came back. And I resented it.

Everything changed after my heart attack. It was instant. I quit smoking cold turkey. Everyone kept saying, "Why don't you try the patch?" And I would tell them, "Well, a cigarette ain't nothing but a nicotine dispenser, and a patch ain't nothing but another nicotine dispenser, so you're telling me to go from one dispenser to another? Are you crazy?" If you're going to quit, then just do it. I will admit that I had a couple of backslides on the cigarettes. The last cigarette I had was about a year ago. No more.

Bacon tastes good. And one thing about pork, it's quite tasty. But I had to quit it all cold turkey. Today my diet is mostly fish and vegetables—stuff that's really good for you. I cut out all the grease. If I have chicken, it doesn't have the skin on because that's where all the fatty grease is.

If you make up your mind to do something—whether it's improving your health or choosing a career—you have to stick with it. Yes, it's hard to do, but it really is mind over matter. You determine what happens in your life. Fortunately, I've always been self-motivated. When I was a kid in the projects in Kansas City, I said, "I'm going to become a famous comedian." I made it, but I didn't say, "I'm going to get a TV show that I hate doing." So I vowed that I was going to get off of that show even if it killed me—and, well, I think it almost did.

I firmly believe that if something in your life is making you sick—such as a job you hate or a bad relationship—you need to do everything you can to change it. Stress and anger really can affect your health.

Fear has never been a factor for me (did I just say *Fear Factor*?). I learned early on that you can't live your life in fear. It's called being smart. You gotta have an attitude. You gotta look death right in the face and tell it to kiss your ass.

I see my cardiologist every 3 to 6 months. I do the treadmill test and run for 30 minutes, and he always tells me, "Well, you have the body of an 18-year-old, so get out of here." He said the damage to my heart happened because of the smoking and the stress. There might also be a genetic link: My father passed away at a very young age from a heart attack. He was 53 years old.

I don't think about the day I had my heart attack. Where I grew up, death and life walk side by side. Every day somebody was dying, so I was quite used to the idea of death. But the first year after my heart attack, any little thing that I was feeling made me pick up the phone and call the doctor. I was doing a treadmill test every month because anything I'd feel I would start thinking, "Okay, what's that?" So I'd go to the doctor and he'd put me on the treadmill and he'd say, "Okay, like I said, you've got the body of an 18-year-old. Get out of here. Thanks for the check by the way." I never felt stupid going to the hospital, though.

Though I think you can make changes that will improve your health at any age, I think it's also very important to educate young people about the risk factors for heart disease. I would tell any kid out there that you don't have to be a Muslim to stop eating pork. It's poison. Put that fatty, greasy meat down—especially if you are a Black male, because you are at higher risk for heart disease than anybody. I think it stems from that diet of fatback having to be in everything. And then I would tell the kid to toss out that pack of cigarettes. Take it from me, it's just not worth the risk to your health.

"9-1-1? I Think I'm Having a Heart Attack . . ."

Of course, we all hope we'll never need to know what would happen if we needed to call 9-1-1 after feeling chest pains. But in the interest of being informed—and of understanding what's going on if you ever need to call an ambulance for someone else who fears he's having a heart attack—here's the step-by-step rundown of what the paramedics and ER doctors will normally do:

- ◆ Upon arrival at the patient's home, the crew will assess the patient's symptoms and vital signs (blood pressure, pulse, respiratory rate). In the event breathing has stopped, many crews now perform endotracheal intubation in the field (placing a breathing tube down through the mouth into the windpipe, where air is delivered to the lungs by squeezing a bag attached to the tube). Alternatively, breathing may be induced by forcing air into the lungs by squeezing a bag with a mask that has been placed over the mouth and nose.

- ◆ Many ambulance crews carry an EKG machine into the home of someone who has called 9-1-1, rather than wait for the heart rhythms to be recorded in the emergency room.

- ◆ If the heart needs to be electrically stabilized prior to transport to the hospital, the heartbeat can be restored with the standard placement of paddles on the chest and shocked into a regular rhythm. If the heart rhythm is too slow (20 beats per minute or less), many EMT crews now carry an external cardiac pacer, which is a pacemaker that is placed on the chest and uses electrical impulses through the skin to increase the heart beat.

◆ One of two drugs may also be used to stabilize heart rhythm: Lidocaine is given intravenously to treat ventricular tachycardia (rapid, irregular heartbeat) or ventricular fibrillation (the heart pumps little or no blood). Amiodarone is a newer drug that is taken orally with the same or better results in establishing a stable heart rhythm.

◆ Depending on the particular geographic area, paramedics may be able to transmit a patient's vital signs electronically to the ER while en route to the hospital. As a result, the ER personnel can begin treatment immediately.

◆ If the heart attack victim is conscious, he may be given an aspirin (325 milligrams) that is crunched up for faster absorption in the body. (If you think you are having a heart attack, take an aspirin after calling 9-1-1.)

◆ Upon arrival in the ER, a heart attack victim is given nitroglycerin through an IV (if this hasn't been provided while en route). This drug is used to relax blood vessels to the heart, thereby providing increased blood and oxygen, which will reduce the angina (intense chest pain) the patient may be feeling.

◆ Heparin is administered by IV to reduce the blood-clotting cells and thin the blood.

◆ ER doctors will have determined by now how much time has passed since the first symptoms occurred. This is the moment when they will decide whether to open a clogged blood vessel through angioplasty (if a catheter team is on site or available to assemble within the hour), or through the use of a thrombolytic drug, or, in some cases, through both. (When both options are available, half a dose of a thrombolytic drug is given. If the blood vessel has opened—this can take as long as 45 minutes to occur—by the time the catheter team is brought in, they go home and the patient is admitted to the hospital.)

—RICHARD KATZ, M.D., *chief of cardiology at The George Washington University Hospital in Washington, D.C.*

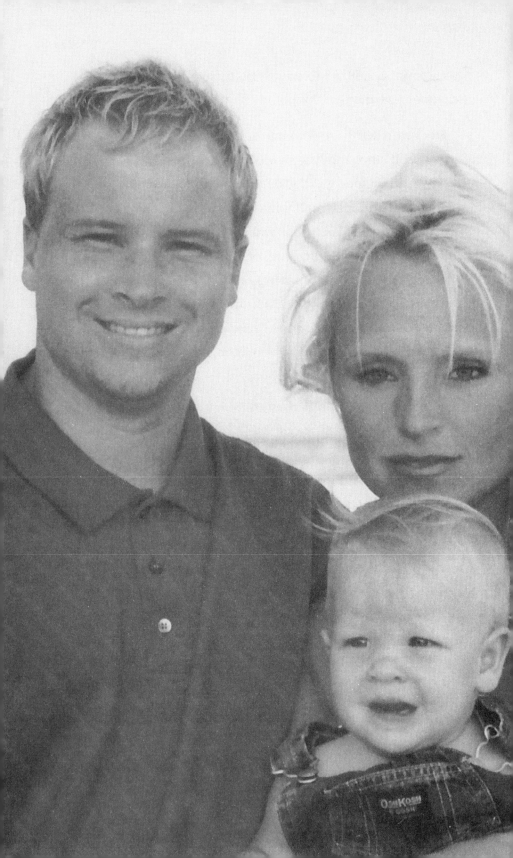

BRIAN LITTRELL

The blond "Backstreet Boy" was born in 1975 with a common but serious heart ailment: a ventricular septal defect, which is a hole between the two pumping chambers in the lower part of the heart. At age 5, Brian fell off a bicycle and injured his leg. The small cut became infected, and when the infection moved to his already weakened heart, the Lexington, Kentucky, youth developed bacterial endocarditis and remained hospitalized during the summer of 1980. Miraculously, he recovered. But when he was 21, Littrell was told that the time had arrived for him to have the hole in his heart repaired. The surgery was done a month later. Since that time, Brian and his family have sponsored a program to teach the importance of a healthy lifestyle to children ages 8 to 12 who have heart disease (or have some of the risk factors that contribute to heart disease).

"I think my heart condition ... has clarified what's truly important to me in life—being married and having a wonderful relationship and having children. ... In the end, my successes as a band member aren't as important to me as my successes off the stage."

I was 21 when I first heard the news that I needed open-heart surgery. I remember that my parents were in the doctor's office with me. My cardiologist, Dr. Tom Carson, said he didn't see the problem getting better; in fact, he believed the problem was getting worse because my heart was now enlarged. He said that if I want to be on this earth another 30 to 40 years and be able to get married and have children—goals that I've always wanted to achieve—he recommended that I go ahead with the surgery.

I'd had this problem all of my life. I was born with what's known as a ventricular septal defect (VSD). My parents were told about it 6 months after I was born. The doctor waited to tell them because he wanted to see how things progressed. When I was 5, I was hospitalized after getting an infection that spread to my heart, which was vulnerable because of the defect. I developed bacterial endocarditis, which can be fatal. I knew I had an infection, but I also believed the problem was going to get better and I would be able to move forward with my life. I had no idea that at the time, my physicians gave me a zero percent chance of recovery. Thankfully, I proved my doctors wrong and was able to return home to my family.

Soccer was my first love, and I wanted to play out there on the field with the kids who were my age. Mom and Dad would say, "No, you can't do that, honey," and I never understood why until later on in life. That's when Mom told me that they didn't let me be as physically active as I wanted to be because the doctors scared them by saying I wasn't going to be as strong when I recovered from the infection. Of course, little did the doctors know I would go on to do 2-hour shows a night and be in the excellent cardiovascular shape that I'm currently in!

The doctors always said that they thought the hole in my heart would eventually close up when I got older. It never did. Every year, I'd go back to the University of Kentucky Medical Center for stress tests, electrocardiograms, and stuff like that, but I was always in excellent shape—being in the band kept all of us in shape. But when I was 21, they discovered that my heart was actually enlarging and the hole wasn't closing up. Blood was passing back and forth between my left and right ventricles, causing a backwash effect. As a result, my heart was swelling.

Ironically, at the time I was told I needed surgery, I felt I was in the best shape of my life. On a rare day off or before a concert, I was always playing basketball. And on stage, we did some pretty active routines. Because of that, the news came as a shock. To find out that something you can't really feel is going wrong inside of you—and it's a life-changing thing—well, that was a tough day.

I had a conversation with the other guys in the band, telling them that the surgery had to take place. But we were so busy at that point in our lives that I don't think they fully comprehended what needed to be done. They knew, of course, that I had a previous heart condition (we'd been together for 5 years at this point), so they didn't have to ask a lot of questions. Still, it was news to *me*, so obviously it was a shock to them. Dr. Carson and my mom and dad and I (and even our band's management) agreed we ought to get a second opinion, so I went to the Mayo Clinic in Rochester, Minnesota. I was given all the tests, and the doctors there agreed with Dr. Carson's diagnosis.

We continued to tour, but I thought about my heart every time I went on stage. Our schedule was so grueling that I ended up postponing my surgery twice because our managers at the time were saying, "Well, we've already booked that time, and we can't take the tour down because it will be so costly." I postponed it for a European tour and then I postponed it for a U.S. leg of the tour.

I know that our management was very frightened that something would go wrong during surgery. Our careers were flourishing in 1998, and it was probably a scary thing for them, but it was just as scary for me. That's when my personality changed toward the music business. I can still remember yelling at the manager telling him I felt like he was disregarding my life when it came to the schedule. Dr. Carson told me not to be pushed into coming back too early after the operation, and so we agreed that 8 weeks after the surgery was the very earliest we could look at starting the tour again. Surgery was scheduled for May 8th, and the wave of Backstreet Boys was going to have to be put on hold for a while.

A Life-Saving Discovery

Once the surgery date arrived and I was at Mayo Clinic, I prayed a lot and I know that my family prayed that I would come through the operation safely. I prayed that I would wake up. I remember telling the nurses to double up on my medicine because I didn't want to remember anything. I just wanted to wake up in a healthier condition than when I went to sleep. I was frightened to death, knowing what had to be done. The thought of my sternum being cracked and my ribs being opened—all these images were coming into my mind and I kept thinking, "That's going to be me." I was sort of having an out of body experience where you are looking at yourself lying there and these people are working on you. I had been carrying around the worry for quite some time.

I remember bits and pieces. I remember taking some sort of antianxiety medicine the night before. Then I remember waking up in the morning and a nurse coming in to shave me—you have to be completely clean. Everything was in a fog. I was showering and then they were shaving me everywhere—and I mean *everywhere*. It hurt, but I couldn't really react because I understood the nurses had a job to do and were coming

PUTTING THE MUSIC ON HOLD

Brian first saw his wife-to-be, Leighanne Wallace, in 1997 when she was selected to be in the Backstreet Boys video for "As Long As You Love Me." They were married in September 2000, and in November 2002, Baylee Thomas Littrell was born. Leighanne was with Brian when he was told heart surgery was necessary, and she found herself having to take a stand when he started delaying the date to have it done.

I remember the first time I ever heard Brian's heart. We were in London, and I put my head on his chest. His heart sounded horrible—it was a whooshing sound. I looked at him and said, "This is your heart? This is what you've been living with?" It was an eerie feeling knowing that he had a serious heart defect.

There comes a point when I think you have to put your foot down and insist that the people you love get the medical care they need. I knew Brian wasn't going to get the surgery done for a while, and when he and his managers put it off twice because of touring, I said, "You know, you have to do this or I can't be your girlfriend anymore." I could see him just putting

in to take care of business, and I was just another everyday Joe Schmo.

There are some other details that have since been filled in for me by my family and Leighanne (we were dating at the his life on the line all the time for work. I told him I couldn't be involved with him anymore if he continued to do that.

It was tough for Brian to take the time away from his schedule, but sometimes when you're in a group, you have to insist and say, "Stop everything. Stop the production." I know he didn't want to tell the management he had to stop for a while because the Backstreet Boys were just huge, and it was one of the biggest tours ever. He didn't want to do it, but ultimately he knew he was going to have to stand up and say, "I have to face reality and I have to have this done."

I have this advice for any heart patient's family: Be the most positive you can be. Ask questions—ask every question you can imagine, even if you think it's stupid. If you're going to break up and cry, go out of the room, do it, get yourself together, and then go back in. For patients, try to be in the best health you can be before surgery. These days, open-heart surgery is done every single day. Trust your doctor, because if you don't, there's no point in going any further. But also remember that your doctor is not God. So if you don't trust him or like him, keep looking. You want a doctor who's sensitive. You don't want somebody who treats you like a number.

time and got married in 2000). Apparently, Leighanne talked with me the morning of the surgery, and I was in good spirits. But when they brought the gurney up to my room to take me down to the surgical ward, I started to lose it. That's when I broke down in tears. I knew I had to get on the gurney and that it was time.

After I got on, I remember feeling them roll me out of the room and down the hallway, and there were flashes of light from the ceiling lights whizzing by. And I remember feeling the threshold of the elevator twice when the bed's wheels went over it—the front of the bed and the back of the bed. I felt that two-time jolt. After we got off the elevator, they wheeled me behind something like a half wall and then pulled me up close to the other side of the wall. My family was there, and I told Leighanne that I loved her and I'd see her in a little while. I told my mom if I didn't make it, to take care of Dad, and I told my dad to take care of my mom, but I vividly remember telling my mom to be strong and to take care of Dad. I knew each would deal with things differently; they are two different people.

The surgical procedure was supposed to last about 45 minutes, but mine went 2½ hours. They sewed the hole closed, but then, in a routine inspection of my heart, Dr. Danielson, the surgeon, picked my heart up with his hand and flipped it over so he could see the tricuspid valve. When he did, he saw a hole about the size of a half-dollar. Later, he determined that that was where the bacterial endocarditis had set up shop when I was 5. It was a blessing that Dr. Danielson decided to check the tricuspid valve because the hole never showed up on any exam or test before the surgery. Nobody knew that I had that hole in my tricuspid valve. Dr. Danielson wasn't suspicious or anything, he just figured, "While I'm at it, let's check that tricuspid." I'm sure it's protocol to check for additional problems, but I still feel lucky. They used an annuloplasty ring around my tricuspid, and they used a Dacron patch and my own heart tissue to repair the VSD, as they had planned.

As I came to, I remember them taking out the breathing tube. They used a tube that was one size smaller than what's typically used for someone my size. I told them I was concerned about my vocal cords, because singing is my life and my career. A big breathing tube increases the potential for damage. But even with the smaller tube, I remember that when they pulled it out, it felt like it came from my big toe!

When I came back into this world, the first face I saw sitting beside my bed was my grandmother's—my father's mother. She was sitting right there, and I kind of went down the line of faces by my bed. The next face I saw was Leighanne's, and then I saw my mom and dad, but I don't really recall getting that far. Leighanne and I had learned some sign language, so I used my hand to give her the sign for "I love you." We have this ongoing joke that I love her more than she loves me, and she protests—and so there is an ongoing battle. So after I did the symbol for "I love you," I did the symbol for "more."

Fans sent all kinds of get well cards. We had the whole room filled with cards. Classrooms sent me get well cards that the kids had made. It was small things like that—just a little message saying, "We're thinking about you and hope you get well and get back on stage because we miss the Backstreet Boys"—that made a big difference. One card, in particular,

WHEN YOUR CHILD HAS HEART PROBLEMS

In 1999, Brian established the Brian Littrell Healthy Heart Club for Kids (www.healthyheartclub.org). The club offers a program focusing on education, exercise, nutrition, and counseling to children between 8 and 12 years old who have a heart condition or are at risk for developing heart disease. Jackie Littrell, Brian's mother, makes a point of talking with the parents and children who attend the sessions. Following is some of her advice.

There are two things I hope every child who is facing heart disease remembers:

Don't limit yourself. And don't allow others to tell you what you can and cannot do. We live in a society where it's easy to be influenced by peer pressure, but you need to know that God has a plan for your life. Brian turned out to be a Backstreet Boy, which was totally above and beyond anything I ever dreamed of. You have to believe that your dreams will come true, too.

Take responsibility for your health. Even if you're only 12 years old, you can still make healthy choices. And by making healthy choices, not only are you going to do better yourself, you are going to inspire your parents to do better. We live in a different society from when Brian was young. These days, both parents have to work, and it's easy to grab some fast food for dinner. But even though you and your parents are busy, take responsibility for making healthy choices each day. Get out and take a walk. Help your parents make some grilled chicken and a salad for supper instead of hamburgers from the drive-thru. By doing things that promote good heart health, you'll not only strengthen your own heart, but you'll set an example for the rest of your family.

To the parents, I say:

Be careful not to overprotect your child. If I had said to Brian constantly, "You have a heart condition so you shouldn't be doing that," he wouldn't have done half the things he did. Try not to limit them emotionally by telling them all the negative things about their asthma or their heart or their diabetes or their obesity. Instead, be a positive influence. Have a vision for the things they can learn. And, encourage them to try new things and to be active, consistent with their doctor's advice.

Nurture a spiritual connection. Keeping a focus on your spiritual and religious beliefs always helps because worry and fret will consume you if you don't have something else bigger and stronger that you believe in. In a way, Brian's ordeal has been a blessing because I see life differently as a result of what we've all been through. Life is so very precious, and the picture today is so much broader than it would be if this hadn't happened to me. Brian's illness put my life on hold and it got my undivided attention. It forced me to focus on the most important things—life and love. None of the rest of it matters. Sometimes, the world swallows up the important things, and you have to have a crisis in your life to get the correct perspective.

stands out in my memory. It was a hand-drawn illustration of a doctor and a patient in surgery; and it was almost like the old game "Operation," where you have to reach into the patient and take out bones without hitting the side, or the buzzer goes off and you lose. There was a doctor's hand in there with a set of tongs like what you'd use to toss a salad. I'm the person lying on the table, and there was an x-ray machine of where my heart was. But there was a sandwich inside my heart! It was like the doctor was reaching in there to grab the sandwich out of my heart so I'd be okay. It made me realize how simple life-changing experiences can seem to a child. I kept thinking, "Gee, how simple is that?" Life can be that way.

When I got home from the hospital, I was still pretty sore, but I would try to play a little basketball in my backyard and walk around the neighborhood. Dr. Carson got me involved in the cardiac rehab program at Florida Hospital here in Orlando. It's the fourth largest heart center in the country, and they have a large cardiac rehab department. I was obviously the youngest patient there. I was sitting by grandmothers and grandfathers who had had double or triple or quadruple bypass surgery, pacemakers, or heart attacks. I learned so much about that stage of life and about rehabilitation. I realized that the older you get, the slower your body heals, and I was fortunate to be going through this in my early twenties. In terms of lifting weights and doing machines like the stair step, I was able to hit my goals a lot faster than people who were older. But the important thing was that we were all, despite our ages, working toward the same goal. That sense of community, shared goals, and under-standing of what each person is going through can be really beneficial during recovery.

To get back in shape for concerts, I needed not only to ex-ercise, but also to sing at the same time. So I would work out on a treadmill or a bicycle and sing along to my Backstreet Boys CDs while I was doing it. I remember one time, a nice lady came up to me and said, "Young man, you have such a nice voice. In fact, you sound just like the CD!"

A New Kind of Stage Fright

We went back on tour 8 weeks to the day of my surgery. I was looking forward to it, but it was also scary. I was mentally ready, but physically I wasn't. I went into surgery at 138 pounds, and I came out of the hospital at 121. I was struggling. We always have paramedics to take care of the fans that faint, so I asked the managers if there could be one backstage in case I needed oxygen. They agreed, and that's what we did for the first couple of weeks that we were back on the road. I used the oxygen sev-eral times—we kept it below the stage where we'd do quick costume changes. It was weird: Everyone there is worried about being able to do a quick change, and all I'm thinking about is being able to breathe. It was a lot to take in, but here I am.

When we came out for that first show, we were in Charlotte, North Carolina. It was sold out. I thought back to the days when I was on stage for the first time as a Backstreet Boy, and how anxious I used to feel. All the stuff you worry about as a new

TAKE HEART

- *Take advantage of the cardiac rehabilitation classes offered to heart patients after surgery. Not only will you be given a closely monitored exercise program and learn tips for following a healthful diet, but you'll also benefit from going through the recovery process with others who understand and can offer support.*

- *It is not unusual for heart patients to become* more *productive after surgery than before they were diagnosed. Being motivated to adopt a healthier lifestyle and set new goals may be part of the reason.*

performer really becomes old hat from touring and touring. Certainly, you're still nervous going on stage, but the anxiousness goes away. That night in Charlotte, I remember that when we called out our names as we do for each show—"Hello, I'm Brian"—I heard this incredible roar from the crowd. I'll never forget it, and that's when I said, "Okay, here we go again."

The will to live got me through this. I believed that I had more time on my clock and that God has bigger plans for me. I believe in enjoying life to the fullest. I grew up singing in a huge Baptist church, and never in a million years did I think I'd make a career out of the gifts that God has given me. To have the life I've had—even with the surgery and recovery—is to be blessed, and I enjoy passing on that message. I think the reason I am here is that I can do things to let children and adults know that life is a gift and what you do with it is very important and sometimes you disregard the things that really matter because you're focused on your assets, or things around you, or your job. It's easy to become consumed with those things.

I'm a firm believer that all the money in the world isn't going to buy happiness or true love, and these are things that people search for all their lives. I think my heart condition has definitely set me apart from the other guys in the band because it has clarified what's truly important to me in life—being married, having a wonderful relationship, and having children. I've got a baby boy and, yes, his heart is good. We did a lot of prenatal testing. In the end, my successes as a band member aren't as important to me as my successes off the stage.

The Doctor's Notes:
WHEN YOUR PATIENT IS A CELEBRITY

By Tom Carson, M.D., of Pediatric Cardiology
Consultants in Orlando, Florida

I'll admit that the first time Brian walked into my office, I had no idea who he was. At the time, he was a little older than high school age, so I figured he was working or going to college. When he told me that he was a singer in a band, I figured maybe he did a gig in some local bar somewhere. We talked about his medical history and about the hole in his heart. He mentioned some of the physical things he did on-stage and how his band was better known abroad than it was here in the States. At the end of that visit, he signed a picture to me and said, "Here, I want to give this to you." I graciously took it, said "Thank you very much," and went home.

When I got home, I asked my daughter, who was in the eighth grade at the time, if she had ever heard of "The Backdoor Boys" or the "somebody boys?" She went ballistic and immediately pulled out one of their CDs, and that's when I realized who had been in to see me earlier that day. So the next time Brian came in to see me for a visit, I brought my daughter's CD in and he was gracious enough to sign it for her.

Brian had some chest pains while on tour, but they weren't cardiac-related. We scheduled his checkups for the end of the day so he could come in relatively undisturbed, and we'd sit and chat. My echo tech would also talk with him. But when he came back for another visit, we repeated the echocardiogram and saw that his heart was bigger.

I sat down with Brian and his family and explained that it's not a good idea to go into adulthood with an enlarged heart. The one thing I remember vividly was telling him this had to be fixed so he can continue to sing on like Frank Sinatra. But he was very worried and upset. The echo pretty much wrapped up the diagnosis for me, and I felt his condition was not going to get any better. And these days, a surgical repair is pretty straightforward. Once you get it out of the way, you can focus on other things.

There were two aspects to Brian's operation: One was to patch the hole between the two pumping chambers of his heart. For this, we used a Dacron patch. But because of an infection he had had as a child, Brian also had some damage to the leaflets of his tricuspid valve, which is the valve that separates the right atrium from the right ventricle. The atrium serves as a collection chamber for blood coming back from the body. When the ventricle relaxes, the blood goes across the tricuspid valve and fills the right ventricle. Then when the heart squeezes, the valve closes and that forces blood out through the pulmonary artery. His tricuspid valve was damaged, and the childhood infection had thickened the leaflets of this valve and made it not function well.

The outlook for Brian is pretty good. Because his heart was enlarged, there's a chance that it may not go back to being completely normal, and at some point he could develop some problems from that. The truth is that surgical techniques and even anesthesia have been markedly improved over the years, and we haven't yet been able to measure how this will improve life expectancy and quality of life for people who have had cardiac surgery. ▨

Investigating the Power of Prayer

For years, traditional medicine ignored or didn't seriously consider healing with what was termed "alternative therapies," despite the fact they have been practiced for centuries. It wasn't until 1999, for example, that the National Institutes of Health (NIH) became interested in funding studies about "noetic" therapies (also known as spiritual and energy therapies), which they termed "frontier medicine." But times change. Today, the NIH is home to the National Center for Complementary and Alternative Medicine.

In one particularly interesting study conceived at the Duke Clinical Research Institute, researchers investigated the power of prayer on patients who were recovering from heart procedures. That prayer affects healing is an ancient belief across virtually all cultures. Yet modern science lacks systematic data to support this belief. In the 150-patient initial study, eight congregations prayed for healing for individual patients at Veterans Hospital in Durham, North Carolina. (With the patient's consent, the participants were given the patient's name, age, and illness.)

Though the study's results did not show statistically definitive differences, they did reveal intriguing trends that warrant further research. While a larger study is currently underway, science still has a long way to go in determining what, if any, impact a patient's spiritual or mental state plays in his or her recovery from heart procedures. Many scientists now consider this a key question that needs to be asked and the answer studied. Because energy, chi, or spirit is invisible and we don't have a tool to measure it does not prove it is meaningless. After all, 200 years ago, the same could be said about oxygen.

In addition, every single person who practices medicine has had an experience where a patient is extremely ill and obviously going to die, but he or she recovers. In that setting, you usually don't have to look very far to find a picture of a newborn grandchild, or a picture of Jesus, or something that gives you the feeling that this individual was connected to something that made a difference in their physiology and outcome. Yet this is not a feature that we routinely account for or measure.

What is clear about patients with heart disease is that they worry about life and death. When a human being is having a heart attack—whether they are in North Carolina or California or India—everything else falls aside, and deep in their eyes is the light of a human being who is suffering and often scared. As we deploy all the best technology, we need to consider whether, or how, health care practitioners might be trained to meet their patients' needs at *all* levels, including the spiritual or mental.

> —MITCHELL KRUCOFF, M.D., *associate professor of medicine/ cardiology and director of the MANTRA study project at Duke University Medical Center/Duke Clinical Research Institute in Durham, North Carolina*

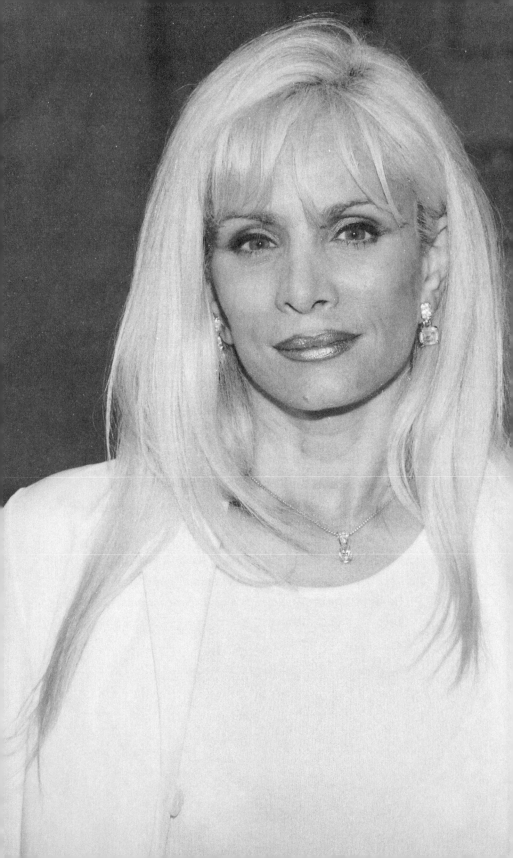

VICTORIA GOTTI

An accomplished novelist with four best-sellers, including The Senator's Daughter, *Victoria Gotti has most recently been a gossip columnist for* Star *magazine. Her father was John Gotti, the well-dressed mob boss who was incarcerated in federal prison in 1992. Today, Victoria is editor of* Red Carpet Magazine, *which features articles about celebrities while they are on—and off—the red carpet. In addition, she hosts a weekly half-hour A&E reality program about her role as a mother, an editor, and a columnist whose daily work takes her to dinner, or shopping, or attending Hollywood premieres with celebrities.*

*"I believe that every day should be unwrapped
like a special gift. In the end, my heart condition
has motivated me to make the most of each and
every day. Each day is precious and shouldn't be
wasted."*

I was born with mitral valve prolapse, which means that the
mitral valve in my heart doesn't open and close properly,
causing a murmur. In and of itself, this isn't considered serious,
but it caused complications when I developed strep throat that
turned into rheumatic fever when I was a young girl. The
rheumatic fever damaged my heart, causing cardiomyopathy,
but nobody knew I had this heart problem until years later.
(Even in someone without a prior heart condition, rheumatic
fever can cause the heart valves to become inflamed, causing
scarring. This scarring may prevent the valves from opening or
closing properly, hindering the normal flow of blood through
the heart.) It wasn't until I was 16 that an emergency visit to the
hospital revealed that I had a heart problem. Still, I haven't allowed my heart condition to change my goals in life, especially
my dream of becoming a mother.

After my heart condition was discovered, my doctors told
me not to get pregnant. Well, to show how well I listened to
them, I now have three boys. My mother always told people

who wanted to ask the obvious but were too polite to do so, that yes, Victoria shouldn't have gotten pregnant to begin with, and was told not to. "But," she would add, "my daughter is far from a stupid girl—she's a 149 IQ, and she's very reasonably street smart. And even as a young child, when my daughter was told she couldn't do something, it's like she was being challenged. She became even more determined to do it."

The first time I learned my husband and I were pregnant was in 1986, when I was 20 years old. Of course, when I think back, I realize it was stupid, but at the time, even if it cost me my life, I was going to have this child. I remember that in the months after I told my parents that I was expecting, my mother would confide to me that my father was upset with me. They would argue about it, and he would say to her, "Why does she not listen? She's so bright in every other aspect of her life, why does she not listen?" My mother just said to him, "John, since she was 8 years old, your daughter has wanted nothing more than to grow up and be a mommy." And so she understood it. She didn't agree with it, but she understood it.

My first pregnancy went full term, but 3 days before my due date, I went into labor and started having contractions. I remember it started out very normally; everybody was very happy and I was in the hospital room being prepped for delivery. I remember the doctor came in and said to my mother, "Okay, we're going to do a C-section because we don't want the labor to wreak havoc on her heart." We were all in agreement that a C-section was the easiest and least traumatic way for me to deliver. Nobody thought I'd be able to carry a baby to full term, but here I was, about to deliver.

All of a sudden, labor starts. Now they're prepping me for this caesarean. They're trying to give me medication, and I remember chaos starting in the operating room. One minute I was coherent and awake and the next thing I know, they're scrambling all around and I'm hearing monitors go crazy.

I couldn't even move my head, but I remember saying to one of the nurses, "What's wrong? Is it the baby or is it me?" She just gave me a blank look, and I remember she squeezed my hand and then she was gone. What really got me upset before I passed out was that I heard a nurse say to the doctor (she didn't even think I was still coherent at this point), "Get the parents in here now because I need them to sign this."

The baby caused such distress on my system that everything was happening too quickly for even the doctors to handle. The nurse flew outside with the doctor and informed my mother, father, and husband that they had to make a choice right then—it was either the baby or their daughter. Even though they were stunned, my parents told me later that there was no deciding. They didn't even look at my ex-husband; it was like he wasn't even in the room. They just said "my daughter." The baby died shortly after birth.

I was later told that my heart had given way at the end. It couldn't handle the stress of the labor, which had come on fast and furious before the doctors could stop it. In addition, I had Rh disease, which is an incompatibility between my blood and that of the fetus. I had Rh-negative blood, meaning that I don't produce the Rh factor, a protein found on the surface of red blood cells. But my baby was Rh positive, which led to further complications.

That night, I was awake when one of the nurses came into my room in recovery. I didn't yet know the baby had died. The nurse asked me, "Do you want to baptize the baby?" and I thought, "Oh, my God. I dreamed all of this. The baby is fine!" I asked her what I had, and she said "a baby girl" with this smile on her face. I said, "Of course I do, can I see her?" She looked a little funny, but she said, "Sure." The next thing I knew, she brought this dead child into my room. I was shocked and started screaming. My dad came running, and when he saw what had happened, he started arguing with the nurse. He said, "Is there something wrong with you? You don't check with the parents first? I told you she has a heart condition!"

I remember after all the melee had calmed down and the yelling had stopped, my father came into the room and sat down at my bedside. I looked at him and saw he was crying. His eyes were bloodshot, and he's not a man who cries. As he looked at me, I asked, "Am I sick again?" And he said, "No, you're going to be fine. But you know the baby didn't live." I started to cry. He said, "You know when you were growing up and I would always ask, 'What are you crying over? What?' And you'd tell me you had skinned a knee and I'd say, 'You don't cry over that because you should save your tears for when you really need them, but I hope you never, ever need them.'" I nodded as I thought back to those moments. He wanted us to be tough, especially the girls. I noticed a tear fall from his eye as he told me, "Well, go on and cry. I'm not going to stop you. This is one of those times." And I never forgot that. We cried together. Boy, did we cry. I was sobbing. He gave me the green light. I could finally cry.

Fortunately, I did get better, and the last thing my parents ever expected was that I was going to come back to their house 2 months later and announce that I was pregnant again. My mother was devastated. I remember her standing by the stove and she was stirring this pot of something and crying. She

PREGNANCY AND HEART DISEASE

Pregnancy places dramatic new demands on a woman's circulatory system. Optimally, a woman with heart disease should discuss her childbearing plans with her doctor before attempting to get pregnant. This advance counseling and planning will ensure the healthiest outcome for both mother and baby.

There are, however, certain heart problems that pose such a great risk to the health of the woman or her baby that doctors advise avoiding pregnancy. These conditions include uncontrolled symptoms of coronary artery disease (angina, shortness of breath); significant pulmonary hypertension (high blood pressure in the right side of the heart or arteries to the lungs); and some forms of congenital heart disease (having cardiac problems since birth).

More commonly, a woman's doctor will be able to reassure her (as in the case of most women with mitral valve prolapse) or may recommend treatment or correction of the problem prior to pregnancy to prevent symptoms or complications. For example, a woman with mitral valve stenosis (the mitral valve has narrowed as a result of rheumatic fever) may have surgery or wouldn't even look at me. I just said to her, "Be happy for me. Why aren't you happy for me?" She said, "Go talk to your father. I can't handle this."

Every pregnancy that I had she went through the same thing. Thank God I had three very, very healthy boys. Each

valvuloplasty (where the valve is opened with a balloon) before becoming pregnant.

Sometimes heart diseases, such as valve problems or arrhythmias, aren't diagnosed until a woman is pregnant, since symptoms may appear due to pregnancy-related stresses and changes in the body. In many cases, this is not a serious medical concern; but some women may require treatment with medication, or in rare cases, surgery, during their pregnancy.

Some medications commonly used to treat heart disease, such as ACE inhibitors and blood thinners like Coumadin, can cause birth defects if used during all or certain periods of fetal development. Some of these drugs are most dangerous in the first few weeks after conception. So before a woman tries to get pregnant, she will need to stop or change her medications.

The bottom line: Heart disease is the number one killer of women. Along with their doctors, women need to take their risks and symptoms seriously, especially during pregnancy.

—SHARONNE HAYES, M.D., *director of the Mayo Women's Heart Clinic in Rochester, Minnesota* pregnancy, however, was high risk and each gave me trouble leading up to, and during, delivery. None of them were caesarean deliveries. I was later told that a vaginal delivery is always preferred and less complicated. The thing of it was, the doctors believed that after my first pregnancy, I wouldn't be able to have children. I spent all three of those pregnancies in bed. With my first son, I must have made five trips to the emergency room in the middle of the night because I couldn't breathe and because I had chest pains and felt lightheaded. So I would stay in the hospital for a few days. It was always touch and go, and each pregnancy was worse than the one before. Still, the fact that I was able to give birth to three healthy children made everything I went through during my pregnancies worthwhile.

A Devastating Decision

In 1998, I found out that I was pregnant again, but this time, it wasn't a joyous occasion even for me. Abortion is not in my religion. It was never, ever an option for me; so while I was scared this time, I felt I had no choice. I was figuring in my age factor now. I was going to be 30, and I just got a bad feeling about this pregnancy. I was so worried that I went for checkups every 2 weeks as opposed to every month.

When I was about 14 weeks along, I went to watch my son play a little league game. I felt a little weird that morning when I woke up, but I showered and got dressed and went on with my day. I was working on my third novel then, so I would bring a little picnic blanket along to the games and work on it. When my son was at bat, I would get up and watch. Well, my guy hit a home run, and I remember jumping up from my blanket. I went crazy and was jumping up and down, when all of a sudden a strange feeling came over me. I remember thinking to myself, "Just let me make it to the car. I don't want to pass out in front of all these people and embarrass my children."

I ended up collapsing about 2 feet from my door handle. Lucky for me there was an EMS worker there, who had come straight from work to watch his son play and had his equipment in his car. I had gone into cardiac arrest. I was flat-lined when he ran over from the field. He shocked me and got a heartbeat again. He called for an airlift, and they transported me to St. Francis Hospital, which took just minutes.

The next thing I knew, I was in the OR. They handed me a sheet and said, "We have to terminate this pregnancy. There is no way. We have to save your life. We have to put a defibrillator in you. And there's no way the baby will survive the surgery— and even if he would, he runs a great risk of being born deformed. And we have to start Coumadin and other medications as well." I just couldn't do it. I couldn't sign. I told them to take the form out to my mother. She signed it without hesitating.

What they had to do was bizarre. I was in a Catholic hospital, so while they knew I needed this desperately and my condition was life-threatening, they had to have me airlifted to Long Island Jewish Hospital, where they terminated the pregnancy, and then have me airlifted back to St. Francis. We landed on the roof . . . I was coherent for that. They took me right down to the OR and put a defibrillator in.

Even before this pregnancy, I was aware of the fact that I would probably have to have a defibrillator because my cardiologist, Dr. Martin Handler, had told me he was concerned about my arrhythmia. He consulted other cardiologists, and everyone agreed that a defibrillator would be a good "insurance policy"—that was the phrase Dr. Handler always used. At that time, he said it wasn't an emergency, but having one would be better than not having one. The pregnancy pushed me over the line to the point where it had to be done.

The next 3 days were a blur to me. It was insane. I woke up from the surgery and started watching a communal TV in the recovery room. I was staring at the screen, but I wasn't completely coherent and still felt dazed. A nurse was changing my bandages, and she followed my eyes to the screen and exclaimed, "Oh my God, that's you, isn't it?"

It hadn't even registered to me before then, but when I heard the surprise in her voice, of course I took notice. They had me all but dead on TV, and the reporter was saying something about "say prayers tonight for Victoria Gotti, who is gravely ill and is listed in very critical condition." They went on to list all my accomplishments—oh, it was horrible and bizarre. Not able to hear more, I just went back to sleep. It was as if I thought, "All right, I'm dying now. I'll just make this an easier transition."

Eventually, thank God, I recovered and was discharged from the hospital. With time and medications, I adjusted very easily. I have a defibrillator that also has pacemaking capabilities, and I barely even have to think about it. The only interruption in my life is that every 3 months, I need to go to the heart clinic for what's known as a pacemaker interrogation. The doctor moves a wand over my heart that downloads information about the pacemaker. It can tell him if I've had any arrhythmia, the status of the battery, and the condition of the leads. He can even adjust the pacemaker's settings electronically if needed. (This is done if the pacemaker isn't responding properly to a change in my heart rate.) The whole appointment takes less than 2 hours.

FROM ATHLETE TO HEART PATIENT

After all that I've been through, it seems strange to think that I didn't even realize I had a heart problem until I was 16 and running track at St. John's University. It was right before a meet, and I just didn't feel right. From the moment I got on the track, my heart started racing. I remember my heartbeat was very erratic; there seemed to be extra beats. I felt shaky and lightheaded and breathless, but I just kept thinking, "Naw, I'm fine—this will pass." I kept on running, which I now realize was stupid of me. But I kept trying to reassure myself that it was just nervousness and anxiety.

After I finished the second race, I headed back to what we call "the shed." My mother had come to watch me, and I remember her looking at me. She had this horrid look on her face. It was an "oh my God" look. I passed by her and didn't even look up to get my congratulations; all I could do was hold my chest and pray to God that I made it back inside the shed and didn't collapse in front of all these people. I knew I was going to collapse. You can feel it. Well, I went down.

I remember waking up in the hospital and saying, "What the heck is going on here?" And I remember seeing my mother, who was crying, and I thought, "I'm in trouble." My mom was talking with the nurses and doctors and I heard her say, "What do you mean it's heart trouble? She's 16, for God's sake." I thought, "I'm in real big trouble." That was the scene I remember the most.

The doctors explained that the early bout I had with strep throat and rheumatic fever had weakened my heart. The damage hadn't shown up until my heart was really tested, as it was at the track meet. I guess one way to explain what occurred was that my body and brain asked my heart to rise to the occasion that day and it just couldn't. I had never had a stress test or any other type of serious testing before. The feeling was that even though I had been born with a mitral valve prolapse, if my heart seemed to be working okay, and if it wasn't causing problems, then don't try to fix it.

Shortly after I came home from the hospital, my mom came up to my bedroom and was all excited. She had an envelope in her hand, and she acted as if it was some sort of consolation prize. She said, "You've been chosen to compete in the Miss New York USA pageant!" Of course, I was surprised and asked how I was chosen. She said, "Well, I don't know . . . they chose you from your photos." I told her I didn't want to be in the pageant, but she just said, "Oh well, yes you do, of course you do." Then she showed me this beautiful white gown. Contrary to what the world believes, my family wasn't well-off; in fact, we were far from well-off when I was growing up. Yet when I looked at this gown, I could tell that it cost more than any dress I had ever owned before. I remember seeing the price tag, and it was over $500. That was just like ten grand to me now, so I was shocked. I asked my mom where she bought it, and she said the name of the most expensive designer boutique on Union Turnpike. I said to her, "Where did you get the money?" She just said, "That's not important." I could tell she had saved; she had scrimped without my dad even knowing because, to him, that would have been a frivolous purchase. When I saw how determined she was, I didn't give her an argument. I competed because I knew how important the pageant was to her.

At this point, I had already graduated from high school. I was in college at 15 because I'm one of those brainiacs who completed all her high school classes before everyone else. They put me in St. John's University because I was already considered in my second year of college. Now, the only thing I wanted to do was finish college, and that was my race. I had been so fortunate to get that jump start, and I wanted to be the youngest student to graduate from St. John's. But after that day at the track, I wasn't able to attend class regularly. So we eventually arranged for home tutoring and home schooling.

Just as my parents worried about me when I was a teenager, my three sons worry about me now. They know that it takes a lot to force me to stay in bed, so if I get a cold and am laid up for a day, I have to constantly reassure them that I'll be fine. I notice that when this happens, they're like three vultures hovering around the bedroom looking for excuses to come in; they'll say that they need to show me their homework, or talk to me about something. I can see the fear and worry in their eyes.

I've found that spending some time alone with each child can help to ease their fears. For example, my little guy always has me come into his bedroom to kiss him good night and talk to him for a few minutes before bedtime. We talk about things that happened to him during the day that he's having trouble understanding. He'll make me come into his room even if I'm laid up with a 102-degree fever. He's not being selfish; he just feels more comfortable talking when he's under his covers and I'm sitting on his bed. It's only then that he can ask without fear or embarrassment, "Mom, are you going to die?" I always reassure him with, "No, not at all," and then he's finally able to fall asleep.

The fact is that my defibrillator allows me to live a full, active life as a mom and an author. And because of the heart problems I've faced, I don't take things for granted. I believe that every day should be unwrapped like a special gift. In the end, my heart condition has motivated me to make the most of each and every day. Each day is precious and shouldn't be wasted.

❧

The Doctor's Notes:
DEFINING CARDIOMYOPATHY

MARTIN HANDLER, M.D., F.A.C.C., Great Neck, New York

When I first saw Victoria Gotti, she was experiencing a rhythm problem with her heart. Her heartbeat was too fast—way above the normal rate of 60 to 100 beats per minute—and she was feeling palpitations.

Victoria's heart problems stem from a bout she had with rheumatic fever as a child. Rheumatic fever most often strikes young people between the ages of 5 and 15, and it's more common in females than in males (we're not sure just why that is). The bacteria enters the blood from infected tonsils, a sore throat, or strep throat. As a result of the rheumatic fever, Victoria's heart is weak and doesn't contract normally. The heart is a pump, and you want it to be 100 percent efficient; if you have 100 drops of water in a pump, you want all 100 drops to be pushed out with each cycle of the pump. In terms of the heart, you want 100 drops of blood pushed out with each heartbeat. But that never happens. The average is two-thirds, or about 67 percent. Anything over half is considered normal, so if more than half of the blood is pushed out with each heartbeat, that's normal. It doesn't become abnormal until it becomes less than 50 percent; it would then be classified as a cardiomyopathy.

Cardiomyopathy is a general term referring to several types of diseases of the heart that interfere with its ability to pump blood effectively and, in some cases, disrupt the heart rhythm, leading to an irregular heartbeat. There are two main categories of cardiomyopathy: ischemic and nonischemic. Ischemic cardiomyopathy refers to damage caused to the heart muscle by coronary artery disease, such as a heart attack. Nonischemic cardiomyopathy can be broken down into three subcategories: dilated, hypertrophic, and restrictive.

With dilated (congestive) cardiomyopathy, muscle fibers of the heart are weakened by disease, though the exact cause is often never identified. The weakened fibers cause one or more of the chambers of the heart to enlarge, and this ultimately weakens the heart's pumping ability. To compensate for its weakened pumping ability, the heart further enlarges and stretches. In addition, because blood flows less quickly through an enlarged heart, blood clots form more easily. Victoria Gotti had a mild case of dilated cardiomyopathy.

Hypertrophic cardiomyopathy is rare and usually inherited. In this condition, the growth and arrangement of muscle fibers are abnormal, leading to thickened heart walls. This thickening reduces the size of the pumping chamber, often obstructing bloodflow.

Finally, in restrictive cardiomyopathy, the ventricles stiffen and become rigid, making it harder for them to fill with blood between heartbeats. This type of cardiomyopathy is typically linked to another disease at work in the body.

The treatment options for the various types of cardiomyopathy differ, and may range from lifestyle changes and medications to surgery or even, in certain critical cases, heart transplants. ■

Living with a Defibrillator

The size of a pager, a defibrillator is a device used to monitor the heart rate. When the heart is beating too slowly, it works like a pacemaker by sending tiny electrical signals to the heart to increase the heart rate. And when the heart is beating too quickly or erratically, the defibrillator will deliver an electric shock to restore a normal rhythm. If your doctor says that you need a defibrillator, here are some things you'll need to know:

♦ The defibrillator will be implanted on either your left or right side near your collarbone (although it can be placed below the collarbone as far down as the chest). One or two leads are passed through a vein to the heart and positioned near the inside heart wall (called the endocardium). The procedure takes about an hour.

♦ You can consider your defibrillator to be an insurance policy in the event of a dangerous arrhythmia. A heart rate that is too slow or too fast can be fatal if not brought under control. Because modern defibrillators have pacemaking capabilities, they are able to normalize the heart rate automatically.

♦ You will carry an ID card that you can show to airport security personnel when traveling. They will ask you to step away from the scanning machines and will inspect you without electronic devices.

- You'll need to visit your doctor for periodic inspections of the defibrillator (or in many cases today, you might need only to hold the telephone up to an instrument that is placed over the defibrillator to collect information). If you're asked to come into the office for a more thorough checkup, a computer will be held up to the implanted device and will collect information for your doctor to review. The amount of battery life will also be measured. Defibrillators have to be removed and replaced from time to time. (This is done in the hospital and usually requires no more than an overnight stay.)
- Avoid arc welders and large electric generators. In addition, don't lean over a running engine, which emits an electrical field that can interfere with the defibrillator's performance. Avoid battery-operated power tools for the same reason.
- Keep your cell phone at least 6 inches away from the defibrillator and hold it on the opposite side of your body from the device.
- You will not be able to have an MRI, though CAT scans are okay.
- Be aware that depression and feelings of physical distress are common after medical procedures are performed on the heart. Remember, though, that defibrillator implantation has become routine, and that most patients go on to lead normal, active lives.

 —MARTIN HANDLER, M.D., F.A.C.C., *Great Neck, New York*

AEDs: When Seconds Count

In 1989, Roger D. White, M.D., medical director of the Early Defibrillation Program of Rochester, Minnesota, identified a statistic that suggested an opportunity: When a 9-1-1 call is placed for medical assistance, the police car usually arrives one minute or more before the ambulance. And if the person is experiencing sudden cardiac arrest, that minute could mean the difference between life and death. (Sudden cardiac arrest is a condition in which the heart suddenly stops beating because of a malfunction in its electrical system.) So in 1990, Dr. White began a program where police officers in Rochester would be trained to operate an automatic external defibrillator (AED), which would now be carried in their patrol cars. Since the start of the program, AEDs have also been placed in fire rescue vehicles.

Today, dozens of people are alive in Rochester as a result of this 4.5-pound unit, which is the size of a hardcover book. The device delivers an electrical shock that stops the chaotic rhythm of the heart, giving it a chance to regain its proper rhythm. And more and more across the United States, AEDs are being placed throughout areas where people gather, including airports and aircraft, sports stadiums, and public buildings. In fact, in 2001, Congress passed a bill authorizing a grant program for states and communities to apply for funding to purchase and place AEDs in public places. Grant funds can also be used to train first responders on AED use and CPR.

Here's what Dr. White says everyone should know about AEDs and sudden cardiac arrest:

- If you suspect that someone is in sudden cardiac arrest, first check if the victim is unresponsive; this is the major criterion for laypersons. Most victims of heart attacks remain conscious and alert; victims of sudden cardiac arrest will have no evident signs of life.

- After determining that the person is in sudden cardiac arrest, do not call a friend or a family member first. Call 9-1-1 immediately because the chance of survival diminishes anywhere from 3 to 10 percent for every minute that lapses from collapse to the first shock from an AED. Our studies indicate survival is much more likely if the first shock from an AED is provided within 5.6 minutes of receipt of the 9-1-1 call. If the shock from the AED is provided more than 6.7 minutes after the 9-1-1 call is received, survival is much less likely. So there is just a one-minute difference between those who are likely to survive and those who are unlikely to survive.

- An estimated 250,000 people are victims of sudden cardiac arrest every year. Of that number, about 40 to 50 percent are found in ventricular fibrillation when emergency service personnel arrive. Ventricular fibrillation is the most common cause of cardiac arrest at the moment of collapse, and it is the only cardiac arrhythmia with cardiac arrest that is treatable with a shock from an AED. The other causes of cardiac arrest are called asystole (the heart has no electrical activity) and pulseless electrical activity (there is electrical activity, but it isn't treatable with a defibrillation shock).

◆ From 1985 to 1990, the rate of survival from ventricular fibrillation was 28 to 30 percent. After 1990, when we trained the police on AED use and increased the number of police cars with defibrillators, the survival rate rose to 40 percent (and 45 percent if the cardiac arrest occurred when another person was in the room or nearby to assist).

◆ Learn CPR. AEDs do not replace CPR, which should be started immediately after the victim collapses. CPR will help to keep blood flowing to the heart and brain and will increase the chance that defibrillation will be successful.

Wherever a community cannot assure its citizens that a first responder with a defibrillator will arrive within 4 to 6 minutes after a 9-1-1 call is placed, that community ought to consider having AEDs placed wherever people congregate in large numbers. To learn more about AED use, log on to www.aedhelp.com or call (866) AED-INFO.

—ROGER D. WHITE, M.D., *of the Mayo Clinic in Rochester, Minnesota*

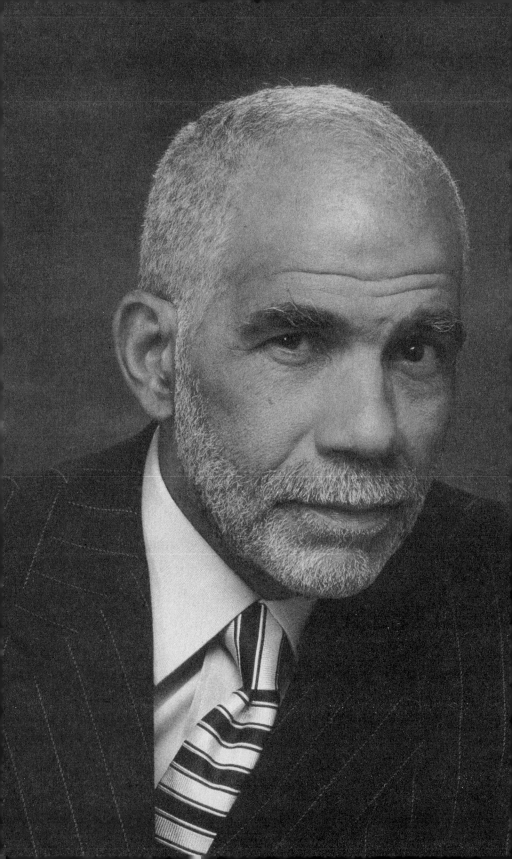

ED BRADLEY

Ed has won 18 Emmy Awards, a Peabody Award, and countless other recognitions for his work in journalism. Today, he is completing his 23rd season with 60 Minutes *and his 11th season hosting the NPR program* Jazz from Lincoln Center. *It was for a story on* 60 Minutes *that Bradley, then 62, interviewed a number of cardiac patients who had undergone unnecessary heart surgery. Little did he know that 2 months later, in April 2003, he would have quintuple bypass surgery that would save his life.*

"I think it's important not to be afraid to lean on your friends and family during a medical crisis."

As I was recovering from a quintuple bypass during the summer of 2003, I watched a repeat of the *60 Minutes* story we did on patients who had undergone unneeded heart surgery. During the piece, I listened to this guy I interviewed say he felt like he'd been gutted like a trout. When we did the interview, I hadn't really understood the analogy, but watching the rerun that Sunday night, I knew exactly what he meant.

In late February 2003, I started feeling a sharp pain on the left side of my chest. My doctor diagnosed the pain as acid reflux and gave me some medication, but it didn't seem to help. So I went back and told the doctor I was still having pain, and he gave me some different medications. This was just prior to the start of the Iraqi war, and I was soon sent to the Middle East. I continued taking the prescribed medicine, but now I was getting chest pains at night. While I was in Jordan and Israel, the pain was persistent and sometimes sharp. Still thinking it was acid reflux, I tried to eat dinner earlier at night and avoided certain foods. I told my colleagues about it because we were often working together late into the night and the pain was obvious. They suggested different kinds of food to eat, and we talked about what I might take or do to ease the pain, but nobody (including me) questioned that the pain might not be acid reflux.

Diagnosis: Don't Leave

On my return to the United States, I went to a specialist and had an endoscopy, which ruled out acid reflux. I went back to my doctor, who said the pain was probably angina; he gave me some nitroglycerin tablets and told me to pop one under my tongue whenever I felt the pain. He also said that I should have a stress test.

The pain was becoming more frequent, so I started doing a fair amount of research on cardiologists. I asked a handful of people I trusted (doctors and medical sources I had) to give me the names of the top two or three people in their profession, and Dr. Valentin Fuster of Mount Sinai School of Medicine and Dr. Wayne Isom of Weill Cornell Medical College were on everyone's list. I had been treated for glaucoma at Mount Sinai and saw a doctor there a couple times a year, so I called him and asked what he knew about Dr. Fuster. He said, "You won't find anyone better."

I set up an appointment with Dr. Fuster for late one afternoon. After he had me do some tests in his office, he said he thought I should have an angiogram. He also warned me that there was a very good chance that it might lead to angioplasty. My soon-to-be wife, Patricia, was with me, and she urged me to get a second opinion. But when I told Dr. Fuster that we wanted another perspective on this before proceeding, he told me that it would be too risky for me to leave the hospital.

I had walked into the place thinking I'd see a doctor, have a conversation, get a prescription, and go home. I had just come back from New Orleans the night before (it was the first weekend of Jazz Fest, and I was planning to go back for the second weekend). My first thought was, "I need some time to think about this. I can't just be told that I need to have some kind of procedure done and that I can't even leave the hospital." Dr. Fuster gave Patricia and me a little room to sit in, and we talked about what we should do and made some phone calls to friends. I finally decided to go through with the procedure, but not before asking some questions.

I barraged Dr. Fuster with questions such as "What's involved in the angiogram?" and "What's the downside?" I had him explain the risks involved and asked, "Are you certain that there is no alternative?" After my questions were answered, I was prepped for the angiogram.

I guess I shouldn't have been surprised that I was at risk for cardiac problems. My mother had a stroke, so there was probably some hereditary basis for my heart problems. I even had a minor stroke myself a few years earlier, but I was lucky because I didn't suffer any long-term effects from it, such as the limping or partial paralysis that's sometimes associated with stroke. It happened when I was on vacation, but it wasn't anything dramatic. In fact, the only change I noticed was that my vision was different. That prompted me to go to the doctor after a day or two. After evaluating me, the doctor told me he thought I had had a stroke.

What a Difference a Day Makes

The doctors went in to do the angiogram with the idea that they would probably also have to do an angioplasty. But when they did the angiogram, they found that my left main artery was 80 percent blocked. Dr. Fuster informed me that I had to have bypass surgery, and it was quickly scheduled for the next morning. The thing of it was, I had been anesthetized for the angiogram and I don't recall the conversation, but I know it did take place. Dr. Fuster asked Dr. Isom to come to the hospital and look at the angiogram, and he concurred that I needed bypass surgery.

The devil is in the details, so I decided I didn't need to know everything that was going to happen during the surgery. I remember thinking, "Let's just get this over with." Still, I didn't sleep very well that night. A cardiac care unit is really noisy—there are a lot of machines beeping and nurses walking back and forth. Plus, I was feeling anxious about what would happen in the morning. I was aware of the operation's risks: There was a chance I could have a heart attack or a stroke, and either one could be severe. Yet as anxious as I was feeling, I knew I had no control over what would happen, which is why I just gave myself over and said, "I'm in the hands of two experts—Dr. Fuster, the cardiologist, and Dr. David Adams, the surgeon—so let's just go and get this thing done."

The next morning, I have a memory of being wheeled out of the room where I slept and waiting somewhere before they took me into an operating room. The next thing I knew, I was waking up in recovery. I looked around and saw Patricia. I think she saw the question in my eyes, and she reassured me that I hadn't had a heart attack or stroke during the surgery. Everything had gone well.

During those first few hours after waking up, I started thinking about how I hadn't been hospitalized before, other than once when I was a child and once when I had a knee operation. I had never even really been sick. In fact, when I got the flu a couple years ago, I remember saying to someone that I hadn't had the flu since 1956. That day in the hospital, I laid there thinking, "How did this happen to me?" I ate well, I controlled my weight, I exercised regularly, and I hadn't smoked for more than 20 years. My good cholesterol was high and my bad cholesterol was low, and I kept saying and thinking, "Why?" The answer I came up with was twofold: I believe most of it is probably hereditary and part of it is stress, which is something I've been under for as long as I've been working as an anchor and investigative reporter.

On the Road to Recovery

I ended up staying longer in the hospital than the average bypass patient because I had a pulmonary embolism. Three days after surgery, the doctors became aware that something was wrong. I was having trouble breathing, but I reasoned that my chest had just been split open and for the past few days a lot of things had been going the wrong way. The doctors told me they were going to have to insert something like a net that would catch the clots. They explained it was a short procedure and I wouldn't need to be put under.

I believe I got through the surgery and its complications because I was both physically and mentally strong when I went into the hospital. Plus, I had a very good support system in friends and family, beginning with Patricia. I couldn't have gone through this without her by my side. I think it's important not to be afraid to lean on your friends and family during a medical crisis. Patricia and her sister were in the hospital with me every day, and it wasn't anything they said as much as it was their presence in the room that made a difference. In addition, I had lifelong friends who came to be with me from Philadelphia and two friends who came from South Africa. They would just come by the hospital and sit and keep me company and share a meal. The flowers and cards and greetings that came in really struck me as well because they meant that there were people out there trying to help me get through this.

I was discharged from the hospital after a dozen days. I remember that the trip home was difficult from the moment they took me out of the wheelchair. Getting out of the car and going into the apartment building was a real effort.

For the first few days I walked around the apartment three or four times a day, and each time was an effort. I do remember the first day that I was able to go outside for a walk. I made it one block before turning around and coming back. That was as much as I could move. Still, it was a good feeling because that was more than I had been able to do in the apartment. That's when I realized that this recovery was going to be a long road. When I got to the point where I could walk a couple of miles through the streets of New York or out on Long Island near Sag Harbor, I felt like I had really achieved something. It was quiet, there were no cars, and it was peaceful.

I've learned that it's important to be patient with yourself during recovery and to focus on the small gains you make each day. In addition to my walks, I had a physical therapist come in and help me do exercises that would make me stronger. I did this in place of the cardiac rehabilitation classes that many patients attend at the hospital.

People sent a lot of CDs, and I listened to many of them as I recovered. I listened to Duke Ellington, John Coltrane, Miles Davis, Ella Fitzgerald, Billie Holiday, and a lot of people I had grown up with. It was like going back to my roots of jazz.

I eased back into work by going in 3 days a week, then 4. It wasn't until late September 2003 that I even made my first road trip to do a story. As I started talking to people about my experience, I was surprised to learn how many other people had gone through the same thing and what their lives were like. There were people in my office who had had bypass surgery that I never knew had heart problems. Talking with them reinforced my belief that this was something I just had to get through, and that recovery wouldn't come in one fell swoop. I'm on the road to a full recovery, and when I get there, I'll be even healthier than before.

Looking back now, I think the thing that was most surprising for me was the fact that everything came out of the blue. Of course, in hindsight I can see that the pain I was experiencing in my chest was a warning sign, but I had chalked it up to heartburn and acid reflux. So, in that sense, I had no warning. As a result, when Dr. Fuster said, "I don't think you should leave the hospital," it came as a shock. A total shock.

Undergoing heart surgery makes you much more aware of

your own—and others'—mortality. When you've rarely been sick, you start to think life is always like that. But when you go through something like this, you gain a deeper perspective and realize the importance of making the most of every day that you have.

⌦

THE DOCTOR'S NOTES:
NO VIPs IN CARDIAC CARE

VALENTIN FUSTER, M.D., Ph.D., former president of the American Heart Association, president-elect of the World Heart Federation, and director of the Cardiovascular Institute at Mount Sinai School of Medicine in New York City

I had never met Ed Bradley before he came in for an office visit, but I was aware of who he is, of course. When he came in, it was late in the day and he told me about some symptoms he had been having. I interpreted those symptoms to be angina, so I had him do a few sit-ups in the examining room—we didn't even do a treadmill test. Sit-ups may seem to many to be quite primitive, but they're a test I use. Sometimes, I'll have the patient walk up flights of stairs in the stairway of the building at 6:00 P.M. on a Friday if I can't get exercise tests and treadmills ordered. As a doctor, I've learned to use whatever I have that's available.

As Ed did the sit-ups, I could hear what I call extra heart sounds, so it was obvious something was wrong. Normally, there are two sounds; one is when the heart contracts and the other is when the valves close. I was hearing three sounds, and this, in my view, meant his heart muscle was suffering. That's when I told him I couldn't allow him to go home. In good conscience, I couldn't tell him that it was okay to leave.

I learned from taking a medical history that he had what we call a hypercoagulative state, which means the blood has a tendency to clot and cause a pulmonary embolus. Most clots are released in the leg and travel through the veins to the lungs. If left untreated, they can be fatal. The fact that Ed had this condition wasn't an impediment for surgery, but it certainly carried a risk.

Two hours later, we did an angiogram and found that Ed's main coronary artery was almost closed. I asked Dr. Isom to come to our hospital to provide a second opinion about the need for Ed to have bypass surgery. He agreed that it had to be done, and done quickly. When I told Ed he needed a bypass, he asked who could perform the surgery, and I recommended Dr. David Adams, who is absolutely superb. Ed said, "Well, I don't know, I don't feel good about it." I could understand his hesitation: I had just convinced him to have an angiogram and now I was trying to talk to him about having bypass surgery.

Ed's case was high risk in every respect. Had he left the hospital, he faced a strong possibility of not making it because of the blocked artery. Whether or not he would have clots during surgery was a secondary issue. The man had an occluded main coronary artery, and it was a matter of what is most important at the moment. We did nothing differently during the bypass procedure as a result of his hypercoagulative state. If you give blood thinner aggressively to prevent the blood from clotting, you may have the patient bleeding from the place of the incision. Ed came through just fine. But throughout the procedure, we were looking for any potential problems as a result of his blood's tendency to clot.

On the third day after surgery, Ed became short of breath. We immediately suspected a pulmonary embolus, and we used an imaging test called a CT scan to locate the clot. We were able to detect it very rapidly; it was originating in the inferior vena cava, which runs from the legs to the heart. Our goal was to prevent a second clot from occurring, so we implanted a barrier, sometimes called a "net" or an "umbrella." The procedure is done at the patient's bedside.

If there's one thing to learn from this case, I think it's the fact that doctors and patients need to realize that all patients need to be treated equally. I made it clear to Ed that I was treating him as if he were any other person, even my brother or sister. There are no VIPs in cardiac care. Had I allowed Ed to go home that day because of who he is or how busy his schedule is, it could have been a fatal decision. ▪

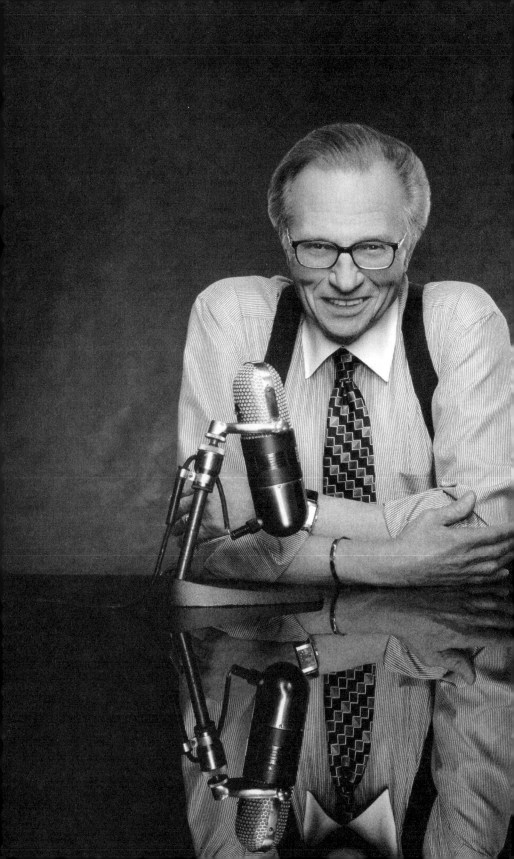

PART THREE

Short-Term Recovery

"The first wealth is health."
—**Ralph Waldo Emerson,**
The Conduct of Life

I t took a while before I understood that someone was talking to me. "Mr. King?" It was a woman's voice. "Surgery is over. It's 6:00 P.M. You have a tube that is breathing for you, and it will be taken out in an hour. Everything went fine. You had a quintuple bypass and you are doing really well."

I was groggy, but I knew I could connect all the dots that were out there. I understood what had taken place, but I was far from being able to comprehend that I'd made it. Instead, I thought of Duke Snider, the former Brooklyn Dodger, telling me his bypass surgery was easy except for "the tube." As a result of Duke's observation, I was as terrified of having the tube removed as I had been of the surgery. But you know something? It wasn't that bad. You know something else? The fear and the accompanying buildup are worse than the surgery. It's a piece of . . . no, it isn't.

By morning, with "the tube" out, I was feeling better, sleeping a lot, and watching TV. My agent, Bob Woolf, appeared at the door and announced, "I've brought a surprise for you." I started thinking, "Gee, Joe DiMaggio?" He opened the door and in walked Angie Dickinson, who I had been seeing for a few months. I think we had a good, albeit brief, conversation, but I'm not sure because I kept falling asleep. Phil Donohue climbed the stairs because the elevators weren't working, and I remember we had a good, albeit brief conversation. Yeah, I fell asleep during that one, too.

Throughout the room were cards and flowers and letters of encouragement from everywhere. Mario Cuomo, then Governor of New York, sent a note saying, "Quintuple bypass? There's a pharmacist in Queens who does this every day." One thing I learned to dread about recovery was laughing. It hurt to laugh, and I ended up putting a pillow across my chest when I knew someone was visiting who was going to start telling jokes. Art Buchwald was one of those people I feared because he started in right away in a phone call:

"Quintuple bypass?" he said. "Larry King needs to always be the center of attention, so Larry King goes out and gets the quintuple. Now everyone has to pay attention." You know something? Laughing hurt, but laughing helped. And with this circle of friends always offering their take, I was feeling better. Someone once said, "He who laughs, lasts." I think there's something to that.

As the days went by, I was aware of the strength I was gaining. Recovery was rapid, and I couldn't get over how much better I was feeling with each passing TV show, meal, newspaper, and, of course, nap. Lying in a hospital bed gave me time to think about a lot of things; one of which was if I ever have to do this again, I'm not going to put it off in the hope a cure will be found or surgery won't have to be done because a pill can be taken instead. I spent 3 months doing nothing but *thinking* about it. Next time, I'll stop with all the reasons *why it can't* and focus instead on *when it can*. It's a preferable way to spend time.

It was important for me to prove I could still participate. I wasn't in any shape to sit in front of a camera for an hour, and luckily, I was smart enough to know that. But I needed to show myself that a "there" still existed outside of the hospital. So a few days after waking up from surgery, I did an hour-long on-air phone interview with Jim Bohannon, who had been hosting my late night radio show. I found myself saying, for the first time, "You know, this isn't as bad as I thought it was going to be." I remember pausing after I said it, thinking, "What did you just say?" But the fact of the matter is, Dr. Isom was right. Once you get through it and begin to focus on being able to walk again, or on reading a newspaper and getting ticked about whatever there is to get ticked about, recovery is rapid. I was proving to myself I could still do the things I had done before walking into New York Hospital, and slowly, I was getting confidence that I was going to be able to do all of them again as soon as I walked out. Participating was important for me, and taking phone calls from across the country that evening was, well, medicinal.

That very evening a lady was listening to the radio show from her bed in another New York City hospital. She was supposed to have coronary bypass surgery the next day. She heard me talk about New York Hospital and Dr. Isom and his cowboy hat and decided if I had made it through this procedure, so could she. But she decided her bypass would be done where I was, and Dr. Isom would be the one to do it. So she got out of bed, collected her belongings, took the elevator downstairs, checked herself out—against the advice of the hospital—and took a cab over to New York Hospital. She told the admitting desk why she was there and said she wasn't going to leave. They admitted her. Dr. Isom met the lady that morning, reviewed her charts, and agreed she was a candidate for bypass, which was done a day or so later. As I was leaving the hospital, Dr. Isom told me about his new patient and the circumstances that brought her to him. I asked for a finder's fee, but he turned me down. That's okay. I was just happy to be walking out the door.

Patients who are recovering from a heart attack or from bypass surgery are urged to attend cardiac rehabilitation classes, but I'll admit I was reluctant to go to them. Both after my heart attack and after my bypass, I attended the classes I had to attend while in the hospital. But after I was released, I came up with every excuse possible not to make the time to show up for rehab. The excuse I used is the one everyone uses: I just don't have the time. It's all a bunch of hooey, but in my defense I will argue that for me, getting back into the middle of things was the best rehabilitation I could have. I already was eating well, I had stopped smoking, and I was exercising. So I didn't want to be told what I already knew. Now, that said, I also know I'd have learned something had I attended the classes. And looking back, I should have done just that. But in my defense (again), I would argue that everyone approaches recovery differently. The goal is to do things in a more healthful way than you did them prior to surgery. I was doing that. End of discussion.

I had also been warned about depression and the potential for sudden emotional outbursts that would come out of nowhere. On a flight to Miami after the surgery, it happened. I just started weeping someplace over South Carolina. The flight attendant came to my side, but I was in such a state, I couldn't tell her between the tears that it was no big deal and I was really okay. It lasted until Georgia. And there were also moments when I just felt low. Everything was going well in my career, but I found myself walking around for a few hours at a time feeling blue. Once, when someone asked what was wrong, I said, "Well, nothing. It's just my spirit waneth." That stopped the conversation from going any further. Thankfully, the sadness and the weeping didn't last, but when they were happening, it was always difficult to try to explain to whomever was in the room (or on the plane) that it was a result of my recent heart surgery.

Even now, almost 17 years since having gone through this experience (and there's a chance I'm going to need surgery again because a bypass doesn't last forever), I'm always aware of any little ache, any brief pain, or any shortness of breath. A few years ago, I woke up feeling a sharp tingling on the top of my ear. I called a specialist in Beverly Hills and got an immediate appointment to come in and receive what I expected to be bad news. The doctor carefully examined my head and neck while I told him I figured there is an artery going from the heart to the brain that must now be blocked in my ear (?). The physician completed his examination, sat down in his chair, and said, "Larry. Your glasses don't fit." The pain went away as soon as a kid with an earring in his nose spent 30 seconds on my frames at the eyeglass store downstairs. Let me put it this way: From the moment you leave the hospital, you are always aware of possible warning signs. That's good, and every doctor will tell you it's good. It's probably embarrassing, too, but quite frankly, I didn't care. If you're going to make a mistake, going to a doctor is a good one to make.

In one of my many talks with Dr. Isom since our first meeting in 1987, I asked how bypass surgery might be done in the future. While he couldn't offer a pill or a cure, he said it is already being done with robotics through three small holes in a patient's chest. Gee, I'm a trailblazer—along with millions of other people who have had this procedure since it was first performed in the United States at the Cleveland Clinic in 1967. (The first bypass was done in Leningrad 3 years earlier.) Today, more than 375,000 heart bypass operations are performed every year. Dr. Isom says he tells his heart patients that it's always better to know him socially rather than professionally. "Unfortunately," he says, "by the time they see me, the horse is already out of the barn. We need to fix the fence and keep the horse in." Looking back, I can easily see how most of my problems developed— genes and lifestyle. I have gotten the message, and the horse is going to stay in the barn.

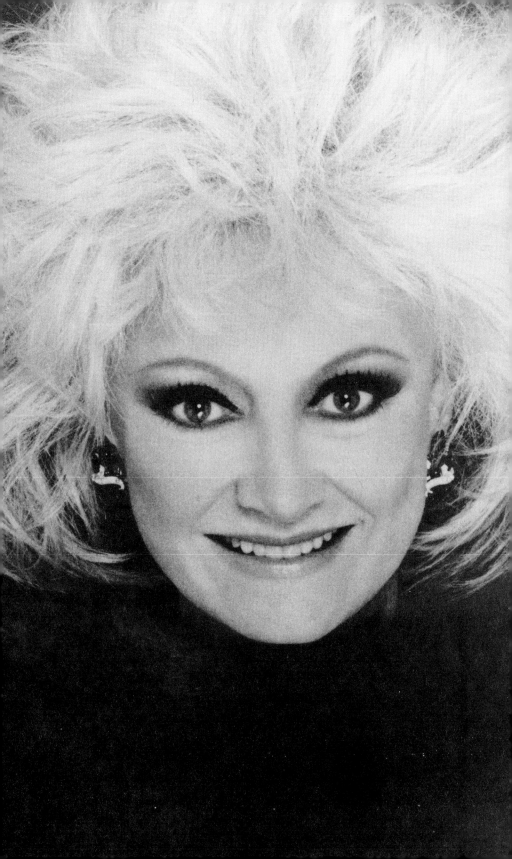

PHYLLIS DILLER

She was one of the first women to do stand-up comedy, and even though she has officially "retired" from making people laugh, Phyllis Diller's trademark cackle and machine gun one-liners haven't taken a rest at all. Now 86, Phyllis opened at San Francisco's Purple Onion in 1955 and later toured with Bob Hope during his Christmas specials for the armed forces. But for a while in 1999, an arrhythmic heartbeat changed things and Phyllis wasn't laughing anymore.

"The best thing for a heart patient is happiness. . . . I am enjoying every minute of my life, and I'm still having fun."

I was angry. I was lying on a hospital bed and I was angry at the doctors. At all the tubes in me. At the incessant drip-drip-drip of the IV just above me.

I couldn't move or do anything for myself, so I was depressed. I have always slept with one of those sleep masks—you know, the black thing you put over your eyes. I started using them on the road so I could sleep until noon since I was up most of the night playing Vegas and doing all those shows. I seldom took my sleep mask off in the hospital, even when I was awake. The doctors would stand there talking to me, and I wouldn't look at them because I was mad at them.

The first time I ever really thought about my heart was when I was 20 years old. It was 1937, and I had to go to a doctor in Lake Tahoe for some sort of insurance thing for my work. He told me I had a heart murmur. Apparently, I'd had it all my life, but that was the first I knew about it. But I didn't do anything differently because of it; I just went on living my life, making people laugh.

I didn't have a sense of anything being wrong until I went to a party in 1999 and just wasn't feeling well. I couldn't put my finger on it—there was no nausea, no upset stomach, no headache, no pain—I just didn't feel like me. I was waiting in the hall wishing my date would hurry up and get me home, and soon he realized I wasn't being myself . . . you know, gay and fun and full of merriment. I was so glad to get home that night.

The next day, I had an early call at *The Bold and the Beautiful*, where I do a guest appearance as Gladys Pope. I knew the layout of the studio because I've made the same trip many times. But I was alone that morning, and I was walking around the halls at CBS and I got confused. I couldn't find the right elevator and the right floor to get off, and I couldn't find the makeup department. I realized I just wasn't feeling very well at all. So the producers rescheduled and shot my part earlier than planned so I could go home.

My doctor has since told me that my disorientation was probably caused by what she calls "a reduction in cardiac output." She explained it this way: The heart needs to pump enough blood to the vital organs, particularly the brain, so they can carry on their normal functions. But my heart was probably beating so slowly that enough blood wasn't making its way to my brain. And when your brain doesn't get enough nourishment and oxygen, you become disoriented.

That evening, my heart started beating 150 times a minute.

I know that because I took my pulse. I could just tell something was wrong. For many hours, it was 150 and I was worried. It's like putting your foot on the gas pedal and flooring it without moving the car. At 3:00 A.M., I decided I had to do something because my pulse was still racing. I didn't want to bother anybody, which, I realize now, was very wrong. I should have called my daughter, who lived only 20 miles away. But instead of calling her, I called a cab. The driver took me to a nearby hospital emergency room. As soon as I got inside, I realized I was going to collapse.

The odd thing is, I was aware of everything that was happening. Each time I lost consciousness, I was aware I was going. Each time it happened, I was sure I was kicking the bucket and thought, "This is it, good-bye." I didn't see any white lights at the end of the tunnel. Everything just went dark. I was brought back by somebody giving me mouth to mouth and paddles on the chest. Later, my doctors told me that I had flatlined.

I had an angiogram, which revealed that I had minor blockages, but nothing severe. I was moved to the ICU, and I remember nurses coming in and constantly monitoring me. I was diagnosed with congestive heart failure and put on a number of prescription medications.

It took a long time for my blood pressure and heart rhythm to stabilize. During this time, I developed a bladder infection, probably from a catheter being left in too long, according to my doctor. Because of it, I had to wait to have a pacemaker put in. (My doctor had warned my family that an infection in the bladder or any other area can feed an infection to the pacemaker through the bloodstream, which could potentially be life-threatening.) It wasn't until 3 weeks later that I finally got my pacemaker.

During much of my early recovery, I was really too far out of it to have even known that anybody had come to visit me in the hospital. I mean, there was nobody home. My precious friends would call every day and my daughter would keep them apprised of what was going on. I wasn't really there.

After I was stabilized and had the pacemaker in place, anger and depression started to set in. I was angry at what had happened to me, and at being forced to lie there with tubes sticking in me. And I was just so incredibly weak.

Three weeks after going into the hospital, I was released. I was in a wheelchair getting discharged when I said to the doctor, "I have a tingling in my mouth, my extremities, and my fingers." The doctor and nurses just shook their heads and sent me home. By the time I got into my living room in the wheelchair, I felt paralyzed. Totally. I couldn't feed myself. I could talk, but I was just so weak. Later, Dr. Fallon told me that I was "profoundly weak," and while I interpreted this to be paralysis (because it sure felt like paralysis), I just didn't have any strength. I couldn't even lift my arms.

I decided I didn't want to live feeling paralyzed. So I decided I just wouldn't eat or drink. I didn't for a few days. But you know what? I got hungry.

THE TURNING POINT

Because I was in a wheelchair, my daughter moved in to take care of me. I had to be lifted onto the toilet. I couldn't turn over in bed. We called my old family doctor and he made a house call. He came over and said to my daughter, "Give her a martini." That was the turning point. He cared. He came by four more times, and he reduced the amount of pills that had been prescribed for the congestive heart failure.

We also had a physical therapist come in three times

THE LAUGHTER LIFELINE

Attitude is everything when it comes to recovering from a medical setback. The attitude each patient brings to recovery is individual as well as cultural. But I find overall that people with positive attitudes who can have a perspective outside of their illness tend to do better when faced with heart disease. These people are able to assimilate the illness into their lives rather than make it their entire life. I've found that there's a direct correlation between how people face a life-threatening disease and how they face other, far less serious, challenges in their lives. People who cope poorly with lines at the bank or at the gas station, or with anger issues, cope poorly with their disease— especially in life-threatening situations.

Comedy has played a huge role in Phyllis Diller's life, and I believe it played a large role in her recovery as well. I think the role of comedy is to allow the individual to stand back and look at what's going on from a completely different perspective. It allows people to maintain some control over their personal integrity, to maintain their personality rather than become

---

a week, and he was trying to get me out of the wheelchair and using a walker. I was in tears every time I tried. I was just so weak. He forced me, and little by little, I made progress.

My daughter would make sure I took all the necessary pills, of course, but she did something that I think was equally important. Every day, she'd lie on the bed next to

a victim of their disease. Once they get out of the "victim mode," they're able to get some space from, and perspective on, their disease.

Researchers have found that the positive emotions associated with laughter actually suppress stress hormones and increase and activate immune cells. And many scientists believe that humor also releases endorphins, the body's feel-good chemicals. I don't think it's a stretch to say that these endorphins are important for the healing process. People who don't want to heal, don't heal. People who have a perspective outside of themselves do much, much better. This was certainly the case in Phyllis's recovery. She has never been a victim to her illness, and she has never let any aspect of her diagnosis determine who she is. She retained her integrity throughout her recovery, and I saw that even when she was weak and tired and in pain.

—SANDRA FALLON, M.D., *of the Preventive Cardiology Center in Santa Monica, California*

me and we'd play comedy records. I listened to Ellen De-
Generes and Jerry Seinfeld, George Carlin and Joan Rivers.
We were looking for laughs. You become an aficionado and
figure out very quickly who's good and who isn't. Joan
is funny and energetic and my dear friend and she really
got me laughing. Joan, God, she's got a rhythm and she's
toe-dancing all the way through the joke. Seinfeld is wonderful, and his material is just so brilliant. Mel Brooks's
"2000-Year-Old Man" was the best of all. If you're going to
get sick, have that video or CD nearby. Laughing is so good
for you. Children laugh 400 times a day and adults, maybe
12 at the most. I'm in the *Guinness Book of World Records*
because I got 12 laughs a minute. Bob Hope went for 6 a
minute. He's the one who pointed out to me the strategy of
timing.

The best thing for a heart patient is happiness. If you're
pissed off, you'll die faster. You may even die over being
pissed off. I am enjoying every minute of my life, and I'm
still having fun. Once it's not like that anymore, I don't want
to be here. I think the thing that keeps you here is having
fun. And eating well. I've always been addicted to three
meals a day—breakfast, lunch, and dinner. No snacking. No
sweets. You won't find little dishes of candy around my
house. Look at it this way, cows have seven stomachs—hu-
mans have only one.

Once I started collaborating with my therapist to get over
the feelings of paralysis, I decided that I could beat the rap.
That's when I said to myself, "I can do this." I had no con-

tact with any of the doctors from the hospital once I came home feeling so weak. I never walked in the hospital. This therapist was a real pro and very religious. I'm not religious, but I could tell he believed I was going to walk again. At the moment, I thought it was great that he was religious and that he thought that way. I didn't. With me, it isn't religion that's going to make me well. It's mind over matter. I could tell he was praying, and that was fine with me. I decided, heck, let him do this his way. He was intense. He believed I could do this. It gave me the chance to believe in him.

On my therapist's birthday, I was so proud to be able to surprise him by walking a short distance with the walker. People helped me practice beforehand. Then I hid behind something and walked over on the walker when he came through the door. He said that was the best birthday present he could ever have. By the way, I have some walker jokes for you: You can tell you are old when your walker has an airbag. When you are a big star, you often have a stalker. I have a stalker, but not to worry. My stalker is on a walker.

I'm doing as well as I can for my age. I've got this rich social life now that I don't travel anymore. And I have my day job at *The Hollywood Squares*, and I do voice-over for a cartoon. Plus, I did episodes of *The Bold and the Beautiful*, and one for *7th Heaven*. I'm working and having fun. I'm not a sit-at-homer. I think as long as you are having fun, you are okay. I believe in nature. A lot of people think you go to heaven. I believe in heaven on earth.

The Doctor's Notes:
SICK SINUS SYNDROME

SANDRA FALLON, M.D., of the Preventive Cardiology
Center in Santa Monica, California

In 1998, Phyllis Diller had two episodes where she passed out. Given the fact that she had another episode when she was in the hospital a year later where she flatlined, it's reasonable to project that she had Sick Sinus Syndrome, which is identified as a pause, or a slowing down, in the heartbeat followed by a rapid heartbeat.

Sick Sinus Syndrome occurs in 3 out of every 10,000 people and is usually found in patients between the ages of 60 and 80. It is the result of degenerative changes in the heart's "conductive," or electrical, system. It is found in the sinus node, which is located in the upper right chamber, or atrium, of the heart. Unfortunately, the syndrome can't be identified through any kind of screening test done in a doctor's office.

In people with Sick Sinus Syndrome, the electrical tissue of the sinus node, which is responsible for maintaining a normal heart rate, slows down and hardens as they become older. And when that happens, one of two phenomena can occur: Either the heart rate will get progressively slower, or there will be episodes where the electrical tissue is even more activated and the patient develops a rapid heartbeat. It is very, very common for a patient to have episodes of a rapid heartbeat and then episodes of a slow heartbeat, which can make the condition difficult to identify and to manage.

The classic treatment for Sick Sinus Syndrome is to place a pacemaker. The device will prevent episodes where the heatbeat would otherwise become slowed, and it will allow the physician to give medication to treat episodes of a quickened heartbeat if and when they occur. Phyllis has a dual chamber pacemaker, and every 3 months it is checked for battery strength. The device should last a long time; the specific amount of time will depend on how frequently it is required to regulate her heartbeat. She still has her first pacemaker and is doing extremely well. ▪

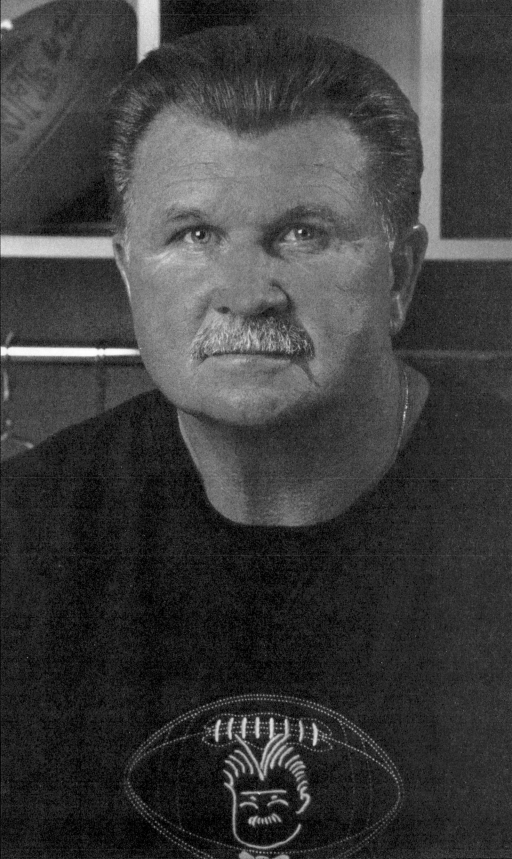

MIKE DITKA

He was #89, a tight end for the Chicago Bears when George Halas was coach back in the 1960s. But by 1982, Mike Ditka was coaching this NFL team, taking them to a 1985 Super Bowl win. Even today, the 1985 Chicago Bears are considered one of the best teams to ever play professional football. And when that statement is made, the reason is always the same: Mike Ditka. He won more than 100 games during his 10 years with Chicago and was the first tight end to be inducted into the Pro Football Hall of Fame. These days, Mike spends weekends doing football commentary for WMAQ-TV in Chicago or playing golf in Florida. He also owns "Ditka's," a popular restaurant in Chicago. Since 1998, he has sponsored Mike Ditka's Healthy Refrigerator *(www.healthyfridge.org) in an effort to make all of us pay attention to what we eat. Ten years earlier, he hadn't been worried about that until, at age 48, a heart attack took his focus off of football . . . at least for a few hours.*

"Forget about the past. . . . Look ahead and concentrate on what you can do today to ensure that you have a long, healthy future in front of you."

T here I was, sitting in the hospital, hooked up to a heart monitor. We were playing Tampa Bay that weekend, and I was told I couldn't go to the game. I felt like I was going to go nuts because I couldn't be there with my team. Of course, I had tremendous confidence in my assistant coaches—there was no problem with that—but I still felt like I was letting the team down by not being there. My doctor had the monitor on me so that he could assess the stress on my heart while I watched the game on TV. And when things got exciting, my heart rate went up. I mean, I get excited and I don't apologize for that because that's part of living. I wanted to be there and I couldn't.

I had been bedridden for 5 days. It all started when I was working out early that morning at the Bears Training Camp. I had just completed the treadmill and stairmaster, which is something I do every day. This day, though, I had a tremendous amount of discomfort and sweat and I was short of breath. I didn't have pain in my chest as much as it was like somebody had put a vise around me and was slowly turning it tighter and squeezing the air out of me. So I sat down for a while and figured, well, this will go away. I had to introduce President Bush (the father) at a rally in a few hours.

Two of my assistants walked in, and one of them said, "Mike, we're gonna call an ambulance and get you to the hospital." I immediately protested. I told them, "there is *no* way you guys are going to do that," but they said they had already done it. One guy told me to sit down and said, "Look, it will be here in just a minute or so." I was still ticked about the fact that they had called an ambulance. That really bothered me. Heart attacks don't happen to Iron Mike. They happen to other people, or so I thought.

If those assistants hadn't come in, I would have eventually tried to get dried off, take a shower, and drive over to the place where I was introducing the president. Somebody else introduced him that day. By the time I got to the hospital, I knew there was something the matter. I wasn't complaining anymore. I just wanted to find out what the hell was going on.

I remember someone saying "heart attack." I didn't believe it. Sometimes, people just don't tell you the truth because they don't know. But then I realized, well, maybe I *am* having a heart attack. I started thinking about the symptoms.

I'd had what I guess were warning signs the previous week when we played the New England Patriots on the road. It must have been angina, though I had assumed it was the result of the cold weather in Massachusetts. I had this sharp pain up my throat and my neck.

I asked the emergency room doctors what they were going to do to help me. They said, "Don't worry, people have had this before and we can take care of it. We got you soon enough."

I later learned that about 50 percent of the people die from what I had. It was a clot in the back right side of my heart, and I was lucky that I got to the hospital soon enough. The doctors used a drug called tPA to dissolve the blood clot. So in a matter of 6 or 7 hours, it was gone.

After the danger had passed, Dr. Alexander sat down with me and started listing the things I had to start doing, as well as the stuff he said I needed to quit. I agreed with him and decided to really work at it. I did nearly everything he said, because, believe me, when you finally realize you're not invincible, it changes your thought processes. I continued working out, which I've always done religiously. And I put down the cigars for a while, though I'll admit I've had a problem keeping them down. I just don't believe cigars will kill me, and that may be a little off-the-wall.

My heart attack was brought about by stress. That's what the doctors told me. At that point, my cholesterol wasn't perfect, but it wasn't high, so there was no reason for what happened except for my lifestyle and the pressure of the business I was in.

Now, when some of the players found out about my heart attack, they raided my office and took all the good cigars. I suspect some of them wished I would have died from the damn thing, but unfortunately for them I lived through it. Still, the shock of the heart attack really scared a lot of people, including me. First of all, you have to realize it was just 2 years after winning the Super Bowl, so the news really took a lot of people by surprise. It was also an emotional time for my family, and it scared the hell out of my wife and kids and my secretary.

As frightening as that time was, I realize now that every day since then is a blessing. I have a friend who had a heart transplant 12 years ago—he's fine, and he still plays golf. I guess we're both living on borrowed time.

After my scare, everything seemed fine. I kept an eye on what I was eating and followed my usual exercise routine. But in 1992, I wasn't feeling the way I usually feel. Something was off. I was tired, and it seemed like I was always yawning. And I kept feeling as though I wasn't getting enough air. I called 9-1-1 (I didn't need my assistants to do it this time). After my first heart attack, I had asked Dr. Alexander if I'd know if it was happening again, and he said three words: "You will know." He was right. When I saw him, I said, "Doc, it's it! I'm having it again!"

I really don't know that I felt the actual attack coming on that much until we did a treadmill test and I nearly died during it. It really hurt, and Dr. Alexander said, "Okay, we have to go in and clear this out." I was happy because I didn't have to have surgery, but I would have if I needed it. I was glad it was just angioplasty. I didn't have the angina like before, but I had shortness of breath and things like that. So, yeah, I knew something was up, especially when I got on that treadmill.

I later learned the attack was in the same area where I had the first one. My right coronary artery was now 80 to 90 percent closed. Dr. Alexander told me if it's more than 70 percent closed, they do angioplasty if bypass isn't needed.

I stayed in the hospital overnight. They don't keep you in there very long, and that's fine with me. The only thing you have to worry about is hemorrhage. That happened to me. I remember wondering why I was so wet down by my groin. I knew I didn't wet myself, so I told the nurse, and the doctors were able to stop the bleeding. This is a risk because you are on so many blood thinners at the time.

I've since learned that there are varying degrees of a heart attack. I always assumed a heart attack meant excruciating pain, but what I had wasn't excruciating pain. It was excruciating discomfort. It felt like my chest was in a vise and it was squeezing the air out of me. I hope I never have to experience the other ones, but people who say they've had massive heart attacks . . . well, there has to have been some warning that they ignored

---

PROMOTING HEART HEALTH
FROM THE SIDELINES

Diana and Mike Ditka had been married for 11 years when Mike had his first heart attack in 1988. Since he was just 48 years old at the time, the news took Diana by surprise. Here she recalls that dreadful day and discusses the changes she and Mike have made since then to improve their health.

I think God got us through Mike's heart attack. We said a lot of prayers. It was such a shock when it happened. It just didn't seem possible that something like that could happen to a man who was so strong and so resilient. To be honest, I think about it all the time because it could happen again, and it could be a major one next time. Even now, when I don't hear from Mike for a while, I start to get worried. He takes care of himself by exercising and eating better, but that doesn't

---

along the way. I just think it's impossible not to feel anything be-fore it. You have to ignore something in order to have that happen to you.

I think you get a whole different perspective on life after going through a medical crisis like a heart attack. You become much more spiritual, and I think you realize how vulnerable you are. I mean, you really are! I think most of us go around for a while thinking, "This can't happen to me; it happens to other people." And then when you or someone close to you has a

mean it can't happen again and be a major one this time.

As someone who has been through this, I have the following advice for the friends and family members of a heart attack patient: Don't panic. Try to remain as calm as possible. And try to be pos-itive about everything. Your attitude really can make a difference.

After Mike's heart attack, I started cooking healthier foods for both of us. We now eat lots of chicken and turkey and other low-cholesterol foods. We've also replaced butter with margarine. And we eliminated some of the things that Mike used to enjoy but that are just too high in fat, such as the egg salad Mike used to love. Before Mike's heart attack, I didn't really worry about what he ate because he was only 48 years old. I know now that heart disease doesn't care how old you are, and that it's never too soon to make heart-healthy changes in your diet and lifestyle.

● *By making certain lifestyle changes, you can actually diminish the damage you may have done to your health in the past. For example, if you quit smoking, your risk of having a heart attack decreases after just 24 hours. Within 3 months, your circulation will improve. After a year, your heart disease risk will be half that of a smoker. And by 15 years, your risk will be the same as that of a nonsmoker.*

● *If high-fat foods seem to be calling your name despite your best efforts to eat a healthful diet, try focusing on eating foods high in fiber, such as fruits, vegetables, legumes, and whole grains. These sorts of foods tend to make you feel full, making you less likely to indulge in high-fat fare.*

heart attack or is diagnosed with cancer, then you realize there are no rules in this game.

The good news, though, is that there are things you can do to try to avoid these health conditions. You have to eat right, exercise, and diet properly. Now I run in the water. I used to run track, but since I've had both hips replaced, I exercise in water, which is easier on your joints. I also try to watch what I eat. (Well, most of the time. Just the other night I said the hell with it, I'm going to eat a pint of ice cream.)

Along with exercising regularly and eating right, I'm a firm believer in getting regular medical checkups. Not getting checkups is like not checking both ways before you cross a street—you're just asking for trouble. If you think you're invincible, then you don't have to worry about it. But one day, you may wish you had seen your doctor a lot earlier than you did. You have to look at your odds and realize that no one's immune.

I think I've mellowed since my last heart attack. I know other people might say "that son of a bitch hasn't mellowed at all," but I know I have. So when I get bent out of shape about something, I just say to myself, "Screw it. It isn't worth it. It's no big deal."

Forget about the past. If you live in the past, then you die in the past. You can change your lifestyle now and you can change things from this day on—but what you did, you did. Look ahead and concentrate on what you can do today to ensure that you have a long, healthy future in front of you.

❦

The Doctor's Notes:
FROM THE ER TO THE FOOTBALL FIELD

JAY ALEXANDER, M.D., of North Shore Cardiologists
in Bannockburn, Illinois

I was pulling into the Lake Forest Hospital parking lot one weekday morning in November 1988 when Dr. John Munsell, an emergency room doctor as well as the Chicago Bears internist, paged me to say Mike Ditka had been brought in with an apparent heart attack. Of course I knew who Mike Ditka was. After all, the Bears had won the Super Bowl just a few years earlier. And as a New Yorker, I also remembered how a certain coach named Ditka had ruined an NFL championship game against the New York Giants. But I figured this wasn't the moment to bring it up.

I rushed to the ER, and when I saw Mike, it was clear from his chest pains and changes in his EKG that he was having a heart attack. I explained what was happening, and he cut to the chase. "What do I do now?" he asked me.

This was a very interesting time in cardiology with regard to the treatment of heart attacks. A few years before, the treatment had begun to change from a very conservative approach with oxygen, nitroglycerin, beta blockers, and aspirin to the use of a group of drugs called thrombolytic agents. The first drug was called streptokinase and the second drug was tPA (tissue plasminogen activator). Streptokinase was the drug used for cardiac infarctions, or heart attacks, and it was very successful if administered quickly. This led to the current focus on the rapid treatment of heart attacks. At the same time, we had angioplasty, which was used electively after a patient was given a thrombolytic agent. Usually, we'd wait a few days and then go in and balloon open the artery. We didn't have stents at that time. The second drug, tPA, was just coming on the market, and we had just received it. I think Mike was probably one of the first famous people to get tPA.

I went over this briefly with Mike; and I say briefly because time is muscle in heart disease and heart attacks, since the earlier you can open the artery, the more likely you are to save the heart muscle. So I spoke to Mike about using tPA and he said, "Doc, do what you gotta do." With his agreement, we quickly administered tPA. Mike did very well, and the artery opened. We moved him up to intensive care and monitored him for a few days.

He wanted to watch the football game that Sunday, so I had him hooked up to a heart monitor. I looked at it this way: If I didn't allow him to watch the game, he would become even more anxious than if he could see what was happening. To this day, I stand by that decision. He got through the game unscathed and, thank goodness, the Bears won. He was hooked to a heart rate monitor and whenever his heart rate went up, an alarm would sound. It went off a number of times during that game. I was on call that weekend, so I went into the room intermittently to check on him.

After 5 days in the hospital, Mike went home to recuperate, which meant not going to work. Well, a day or two passed and he called me up and said he wanted to go to the office, but he wouldn't do anything. I said that was fine. A day or so later he called me again and asked, "Doc, can I go to the football game in Washington, D.C.?" I said, "If you sit in the press box and don't go on the field, it's okay." The next day I got a call from Mike McCaskey, the owner of the Bears, who told me that Mike had just given a little news conference and said he would be on the field for the game!

I called Mike and he said, "Doc, there are a lot of stairs to go up to the press box. If I can just go right to the field, I can sit there and we don't have a problem." So, I'm trying to balance my patient's goals with my need to provide good medical care and I said, "Okay, but *sit on the bench.*" Later, I got another phone call from Mike McCaskey who said, "Look, you gotta be there with Mike."

It just so happened that I already had a prepaid roundtrip airplane ticket to D.C. for that weekend because that's where—

get this—the annual meeting of the American Heart Association was going to be held. So I agreed to go to the game, and someone picked me up at the airport and took me to RFK Stadium.

It was warm that day, and Mike was wearing a heavy Bears sweater. About 4 minutes before halftime he came up to me and said, "I'm not feeling well." That was my worst nightmare. He told me he was feeling lightheaded and dizzy. We sat down, and I took his pulse. It was a little low, but nothing to be concerned about. I asked him if he thought he could make it to halftime and he said yes, so we walked together to the locker room. It turned out that the medication he was on has a tendency to drop blood pressure a bit, and he was sweating from the heat. He felt okay for the rest of the game.

The next day, I was criticized in the press for allowing Mike to be back at work just a week and a half after his heart attack. But honestly, I believe it was something Mike had to do. When you know that the artery is open and you know that the person is doing well, is there a risk to letting that person go back to work early? I think what we have since proven is that with early intervention, either by angioplasty or by the use of thrombolytics, you can get patients back to work quickly and back to a normal, functional life. Today, interestingly enough, this is what happens routinely.

I traveled with Mike to a number of games. But on the fourth week, which was a Monday night game in L.A., he asked me if I was going to be there and I said, "Mike, I have to work." He was a little unhappy (and you can always tell when Mike is unhappy). So I talked to him, trying to figure out what was going on. He said, "I think I'm becoming a hypochondriac. I feel this, I feel that." What Mike was experiencing is common. There is a sense of vulnerability after a heart attack, and you begin to think every sensation could be a sign of another one. A heart attack is an eye-opener. You notice everything you feel in your chest. I call it becoming "cardiac conscious"—you're aware of how fast your heart is pumping every time you get into or out of bed.

Mike went to cardiac rehabilitation classes religiously. This is where patients who have gone home from the hospital learn about exercises, diet, and lifestyle changes. I believe that every patient who has had a heart attack, or some type of surgical intervention like angioplasty, ought to go to these classes. I force my patients to go to cardiac rehabilitation classes because I think it's part of their treatment, like putting them on a cholesterol drug or aspirin. They do it for 10 to 12 weeks, whether they like it or not.

As a doctor, I know I'm not going to change a person's human nature. But when a heart attack occurs, I always see a few common elements, and Mike was no different: Patients have a degree of fear, then some denial, and later there's an understanding of why lifestyle changes are necessary. It can be very difficult to look outwardly normal but know you have a disease that is the most common cause of death in the United States. The interesting part of all of this is that it doesn't make any difference if you are a slight person who tends to be very fearful or if you're a tough Hall of Fame football tight end like Mike Ditka. Heart disease is scary, but as Mike has shown, with proper treatment and preventive measures, you can go on to live a healthy, productive life. ■

Cardiac Rehabilitation Classes

For many cardiac patients, an important part of recovery means a return to the classroom. Patients who have had a heart attack, angioplasty, or bypass surgery are usually strongly encouraged by their doctors to enroll in cardiac rehabilitation classes. In some instances, patients with heart failure will also attend. A few cardiologists go a step further and *insist* their patients attend the classes, which typically are informal meetings where patients learn about healthful diets, begin an appropriate exercise program, and discuss common experiences the class members have shared since learning that they have heart disease. Cardiac rehabilitation programs may be run by a team of health professionals including nutritionists, nurses, or other health care specialists and usually consist of three phases:

Phase 1: This phase lasts a few days while the patient recovers in the hospital. It includes low-impact exercise such as walking in the halls and climbing stairs, as well as some general instruction about necessary changes in lifestyle.

Phase 2: This is a closely monitored 12-week or 36-session program. Patients are educated about ways to modify their risk factors and will complete more vigorous exercise such as workouts on a treadmill, rowing machine, and stairmaster. The patient's blood pressure and pulse are monitored, and an EKG is taken during the exercises. Each session typically lasts an hour. Most insurance plans cover phases 1 and 2.

Phase 3: Patients continue to exercise as before, but without the EKG monitoring. Upon completing this phase, many patients continue exercise programs on their own.

Doctors have learned that one of the most important benefits of all three phases is the interaction among the class participants. By sharing their setbacks and accomplishments, patients have an easier time not only meeting their physical needs—such as adopting an improved diet and following an exercise program—but also overcoming psychological barriers to leading a safe and independent life.

—JAY ALEXANDER, M.D., *of North Shore Cardiologists in Bannockburn, Illinois*

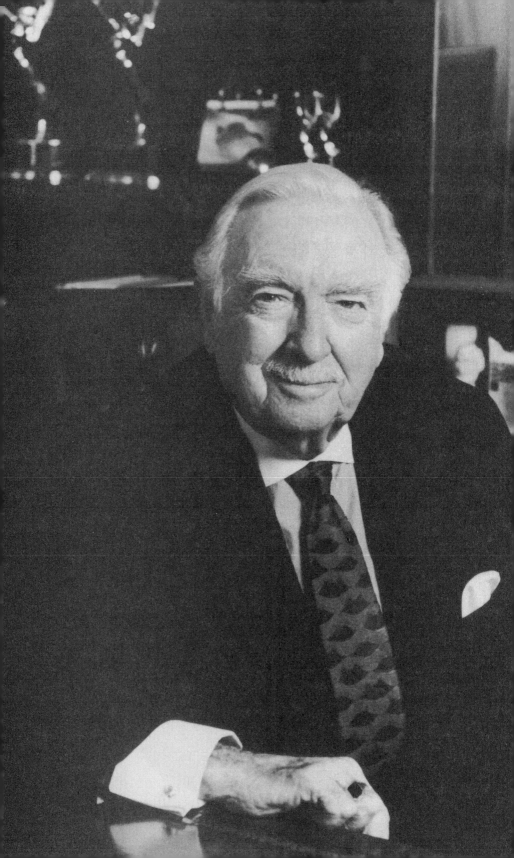

WALTER CRONKITE

*Even though he's officially in retirement after
19 years as anchor of the* CBS Evening News,
Walter Cronkite *has continued to work. He
recently hosted* "Cronkite Remembers," *a
series of news-driven documentaries made for
the Discovery Channel. And in August 2003,
he began writing a weekly syndicated column,*
"And That's the Way I See It," *for King Features. Considered to be the most trusted man
in America, Walter Cronkite has spent more
than 60 years covering wars, assassinations,
political conventions, and other news around
the world. But in 1997, having just completed a book tour to promote his autobiog-
raphy,* A Reporter's Life, *Cronkite started
feeling poorly. His doctors determined that
their 80-year-old patient was in need of heart
surgery. On April 1, 1997, Walter Cronkite
underwent quadruple bypass surgery, which
was performed by Dr. Wayne Isom, who has
also operated on David Letterman, Charlie
Rose, Isaac Stern, and, of course, Larry King.*

*"I think I came through [heart surgery] because I
wanted to. I expected to make a full recovery
and go on living an active and productive life.
I think a positive attitude can make a huge
difference."*

I recall my first walk outside by myself a few weeks after being discharged from the hospital as being the moment when I first felt extremely good after my quadruple bypass surgery. My wife and I had just moved into our apartment in New York City. It looks down on the United Nations park and gardens, which at that time were open to the public with a riverfront walk. I was so delighted to be out there on my own taking my walks as my doctors had directed, up and down that riverside walk. It was then that I saw the light of day. Up until that time, I had this sense of being an invalid in the recovery process. But when I got outside, I realized I was on my own again, and that the recovery was complete as far as I was concerned— although my doctors were still directing me in all kinds of exercises and that sort of thing. This was the independence I was depending upon, and it came a little earlier than I expected.

The first hint that something might be wrong with my heart came when I was about to go on a trip to the Far East with my wife, and I felt a little discomfort in my upper chest. I thought,

"Well, if I'm going on this trip, I better have it checked out before I go." I also had been feeling a tightening in my chest at night. If I hadn't been about to go on a trip, I wouldn't have gone to the doctor's office at all.

Even when I went in for the office visit, I didn't think it was anything that serious. I was very active until that point and had no idea whatsoever that I had a heart problem. I played a lot of tennis and did a lot of walking, so I was dumbfounded when my doctor said, "We've got a problem here." And when he first mentioned that bypass surgery might be in my future, I was shocked. My first reaction was "Oh, @#$&."

Our family doctor is a cardiologist of some world renown. As a matter of fact, he teaches and conducts various seminars and conferences for other doctors. He sent me to Dr. Wayne Isom for a second opinion on the best way to proceed. At this point, the doctors were contemplating whether to do an angioplasty or bypass surgery. They determined that I had what is known as left main stem blockage, and that makes angioplasty more dangerous. Plus, I was having nocturnal angina, meaning the discomfort was waking me up at night. Dr. Isom thought this was a bad sign, since it meant I was feeling discomfort even when I wasn't doing anything physical. The group agreed that a bypass was necessary, and I agreed to it, of course. I had faith in my regular doctor and, after meeting Dr. Isom, I had faith in him, too.

When I sat down with Dr. Isom, I did my usual grilling. I do that every time I consult a doctor, even when I just have a cold, and I think it's something every patient should do. I went through the details of what would happen as thoroughly as I felt I could. I don't think I went through it nearly as thoroughly as my family thought I should have, though. They were asking more questions of me than I had asked of the doctor. And I couldn't answer most of them. But I don't recall feeling serious trepidation. I thought I was in good hands. The doctors knew what they were doing, and they convinced me that they do this all the time. They also convinced me that I wasn't in critical shape. I don't really think I bore any great concern that I wasn't going to be okay. So there wasn't any moment when I said, "Thank God, I'm going to make it." That just didn't happen.

We set April 1st as the date for the procedure. I'm sure there were comments made about it since that's April Fool's Day, but I can't remember any of them now. When I woke up after the procedure, I do think I was pleased that I was in no more discomfort. But for me, the absolute worst part was the intensive care unit. That was a brutal 3 or 4 days.

You are under constant surveillance when you're in the ICU. I remember the door being kept open and hearing everything that was taking place outside in the noisy hall—the constant attention, people poking you, taking your temperature, taking your pulse, and all that sort of thing over and over and over again—right through the night so you couldn't get a good night's sleep. And it's not a very comfortable room. They're as close to wards as you can get without it being a ward. It was just a frightful experience. I was ready to leave. If I could have walked out of that intensive care unit, I was prepared to get up and run. I was quite ready to be discharged. I had no trepidation about leaving.

Except for those couple of nights in intensive care, I handled the operation well. I think I came through it because I wanted to. I expected to make a full recovery and go on living an active and productive life. I think a positive attitude can make a huge difference.

My recovery was quite simple. I really did exceedingly well. I think Dr. Isom felt the same way. I was discharged from the hospital at the expected time; I was not delayed in that at all. There weren't any medical setbacks. The only thing that didn't go according to plan was that I wasn't able to go home after leaving the hospital because we were in the middle of moving out of our house. Our furniture was being moved out of the old house, but our apartment wasn't quite ready, so we had to go to a hotel for the first week or two of my recovery. We had hotel service, but I didn't have a nurse on a full-time basis. Visiting nurses were coming in a couple of times a day and checking on me. But otherwise it was a very, very simple recovery for me—absolutely no complications of any kind, and no sense on my part that there were any problems. I was up and walking the halls of the hotel, getting my exercise on schedule, and was very pleased with the way that went. My recovery was quite quick.

I believe that a sense of humor is essential. I think the long face and down-in-the-mouth kind of approach is not appealing at all. I would find that disconcerting. Dr. Isom gives you a sense that all is right with the world. He has an absolutely supreme bedside manner. While he's serious in telling you the diagnosis and what needs to be done, at the same time he has a great sense of humor. And he exudes confidence, which is what you need, I suppose, in this kind of situation.

The surgery didn't seem to affect me psychologically at all. I know that my cardiologist said doctors have written entire books on the psychological reaction to heart surgery, and how prevalent it is, but I had absolutely no depression or emotional upset of any kind. He was rather surprised and asked me questions about it, but I just never thought anything of that kind. It was an operation that had to be done, we did it, and I recovered well.

I looked at surgery as something that was necessary, though I was disturbed that it was interrupting my life. With me, the surgery was nothing more than an annoyance. The doctors kept emphasizing the routine nature of what was to happen during the operation. Rather than worrying about how the surgery would go, my concern was with whether I would be equally as active when I came out of this thing as when I went in. The doctors assured me that they expected me to make a full recovery, and I'm happy to say that their prediction came true.

〜◇〜

The Doctor's Notes:
UNDERSTANDING BYPASS SURGERY

O. WAYNE ISOM, M.D., chairman of cardiothoracic surgery at
Weill Cornell Medical College in New York City

Despite all the advanced testing techniques that are available to me as a heart surgeon, there are simply some things about bypass surgery I can't predict until I'm actually in the operating room. For example, prior to surgery, I will never tell a patient how many bypasses they need because I won't know until I go in. Each of us has three vessels supplying the heart (the right coronary artery, the left anterior descending, and the left circumflex). But no two people's vessels look the same. You may have one vessel with a blockage in it, and that vessel may have two large branches with blockages in them; so to get that one vessel bypassed, it may take three separate bypasses to re-establish flow there. Or you may have just one vessel with a blockage, and all you need is one bypass to fix it. So it all varies depending on the branching of the vessels.

In addition, the vessel needs to be a millimeter or bigger in diameter to accept a graft; if it's smaller, I'll likely leave it alone. The thing that determines how many bypasses I'll do is the status of the vessel out beyond the blockage—how badly diseased it is, or if it's large enough that I can get a graft into it. The angiogram tells me that the vessel is blocked, and I'll develop a plan based on what I see in the angiogram. But it's not until I get in there and can evaluate the vessel head-on that I decide whether it should be considered for bypass. Approximately 10 percent of the time, once I'm actually inside the patient I'll need to alter the plan I developed based on the angiogram.

It's important to realize that the number of bypasses performed doesn't indicate the degree of illness. In fact, the person who has two bypasses may be in a lot worse shape than the person who has five. A person could even have as many as nine or ten bypasses. The most I've ever done is eight, but those are decisions you make when you get there.

Statistics show a promising trend as far as when bypass surgery is usually needed: In the early 1970s, the mean age of men having bypass surgery was 52, and for women it was 56. In 2001, the mean age for both was 77. Surgery is occurring later for cardiac patients because medicine is identifying risk factors earlier, while providing improved treatment techniques. ■

FIVE QUESTIONS TO ASK
YOUR CARDIOLOGIST

When I meet with cardiac patients prior to surgery, I always tell them success is dependent on their participation. If the patient is having bypass surgery, I make the point that this procedure is not a cure; it is a repair. The patient is going to have to do things to make sure this doesn't happen again. This also means he'll need to ask questions. Here are five that need to be part of a conversation with your doctor:

1. *What are my chances at this institution?* If your doctor has done only a small number of these procedures, you should find someone with more experience.

2. *What are specific issues for me?* Put it simply by saying, "Tell me about me." Find out if there are particular issues that are unique to your situation. If there are, ask what specific things you need to do to address these issues.

3. *What medications will I be given?* Prior to your surgery, ask what each pill or medication is before you take it. Be clear on what it is supposed to do. There are cases where a patient is inadvertently given the wrong medicine, and this is one more check and balance to ensure that this doesn't happen to you. After surgery, ask the same questions.

4. *What do I need to do in the post-operative period to get back on my feet?* Find out what sorts of exercise will

be appropriate for you, and get a list of activities that you shouldn't attempt. Ask about the potential of depression after surgery and how best to handle it. And find out about the changes you should be making in your diet as each week passes after your hospital release.

5. *What is it that I need to do differently?* You should know your blood pressure and cholesterol numbers as well as you know your social security number. Be aware of the role these have in your health. You want to do everything possible to make sure you won't need cardiac surgery again.

—FRANK SMART, M.D., *medical director of advanced heart failure/cardiac transplantation at the Texas Heart Institute at St. Luke's Episcopal Hospital in Houston*

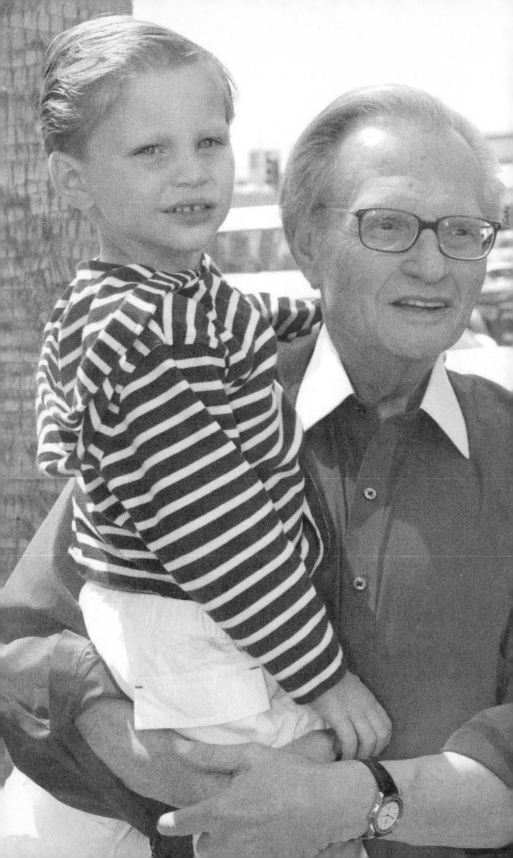

PART FOUR

Surviving and Thriving

"Give a man health and a course to steer and he'll never stop to trouble about whether he's happy or not."
—George Bernard Shaw

April 2004

In the years that have passed since I walked into the emergency room of George Washington University Hospital, I have come to believe there is something to be said for being "scared straight." Fear can be a good teacher, and that's what it took for me to become a good student. But I also understand that because everyone is different, there is no single, correct way to handle this chronic disease of the heart, as evidenced by the stories you've been reading. Despite all the big words and medical techniques and teams involved, it's a personal thing. As a result, each of us will recover from heart disease in a different way, and what works for one isn't necessarily going to be the ticket for another.

Maybe it's because I have a Type A personality or maybe it's something else, but even today I make no attempt to avoid talking about what happened. Yes, there are times when someone will say, "Larry, will you please just shut up about The

Heart for a while?" (or a variation on that theme with more colorful language). I don't start conversations with the topic, but if I'm at a party and someone asks, "How do you feel?" well, that's an open door. I've come to learn that being scared straight isn't a momentary thing; it stays with you as long as you need it. In my case, that's going to be for the rest of my life.

Hospital staffs have asked me to talk with patients prior to their having bypass surgery, and when I have the time, I do just that. I always tell them "as scared as you are the night before, you'll be amazed at how much better you feel every day after surgery. It seems impossible, but it can be a walk in the park." Yes, I tell them it's a piece of cake. But it's only a piece of cake when you have some distance from that horrible night before surgery and the days that led up to it.

Still, for others who have been through that first terror—that time when fear starts running the show, when you see an emergency room while on your back on a gurney, when you hear the word "surgery" as a guy in a white coat looks at you—sometimes the last thing those folks want to do is talk about it. So I understand the differences in how each of us handles experiences like this. My conclusion: There is no one right way to move from the "Oh, @#$&!" stage to the "Where do I go from here?" stage. For most of us, getting back into a routine and making good with The Schedule is a way to get from one to the other. Talking about it works for me, but there are many who choose to put the surgery and days of recovery behind them and quietly move on to the next event. Some people have said they worry that a board of directors or a producer or just a plain old boss will now see them as damaged goods. It's illegal, but that doesn't mean it can't happen, and that's another reason they choose to be low key.

After my bypass surgery, I had a call from my brother Marty, who told me about the chest pains he had been having. Considering the way the past year had turned out for me, Marty knew all too well that our family's genes were a major risk factor for heart disease. He saw a cardiologist and was told he needed an angioplasty. When it became obvious the artery was clotting up again, he was told that a bypass was the next step. To his credit, Marty didn't wait 3 months to have the surgery, like his brother did. As soon as he understood what had to be done, he made arrangements to meet Dr. Isom "professionally." He had his bypass exactly 6 months from the day I had mine. No, don't read anything into that—although heart disease does make you think a little longer about conspiracy theories, especially if you have genes that leave you vulnerable to cardiac problems.

Marty and I spoke at length prior to his surgery about how to prepare, what to be thinking about, and how, if our father had lived during these times, he might have been around longer than his 43 years. I told him that in the back of my mind, I had always thought I'd be dead at age 43, too. So when I hit 44, I started thinking, "I'm not going to die from any disease." Yeah, I know.

We talked about getting ready, and I suggested that he not have his kids with him the night before surgery because once you see them and then say good-bye, you spend the rest of the night wondering if you've just seen them for the last time. My kids were at my bedside the night before my bypass, and after they left, I was focused on the very real possibility that this could be it. Had we said our last good-bye? Marty made the right decision: His kids weren't even in the hospital the day before he had his surgery.

Thankfully, Marty recovered and returned to work. We talk more now than we did when we grew up together on 83rd Avenue in Brooklyn. The experience pulls you closer to others. It's the result, I guess, of being vulnerable and, maybe most important, of knowing the whole shebang can end at any moment. I think that's what happens when you become a student—the learning occurs in just seconds, but the lesson takes years to fully comprehend.

Looking back, the summer of 1988 was all politics. The Democrats held their political convention in New Orleans, where George H. W. Bush had just picked Indiana Senator Dan Quayle as his running mate against Massachusetts Governor Michael Dukakis and Texas Senator Lloyd Bentsen. It had been about 9 months since my surgery, and I was walking every day and avoiding the New Orleans cuisine; instead, I would choose sliced turkey in a salad with just a little olive oil and vinegar. That was it. Skim milk with coffee and not much more. I had built up confidence that I was going to be able to keep hosting both my television and radio shows (the radio time had been cut to 3 hours a night), and I felt good—even without a beignet for breakfast or gumbo for lunch.

Dick Cheney, who at the time was a Wyoming congressman, had been booked as a guest on my TV show one evening during the convention. Unlike the way I've known him to work in earlier interviews (usually he arrives as the introduction to the show is playing), he arrived 15 minutes ahead of schedule, saying he wanted to talk with me someplace quiet before we went on the air. So we walked into a stairwell of the massive New Orleans Superdome, and I hoped I was going to be tipped off to something that would be a big news story. Well, it was and it wasn't. He told me he was leaving the following morning to have bypass surgery back in Washington, D.C., and he wanted to know what to expect.

"If you look at what they want to do, there is no way it should work," I admitted. "There isn't anything logical about it at all, but you know what? . . ."

Cheney didn't say anything. I waited, but he just looked at me.

"It's a piece of cake," I said. He told me everyone tells him that. We went on the air and he answered all the questions, but during that interview, both of us, I think, were focused on things nonpolitical. He underwent successful quadruple bypass surgery 2 days later and has gone on to even bigger things professionally, though he has suffered four heart attacks in his life and now has a pacemaker.

The thing about having any kind of chronic disease is the fact that you never get a day off. I remember having dinner one evening with a television anchorwoman who is diabetic. She excused herself from the table as her stone crab entrée was set down so that she could inject the required dose of insulin prior to eating. When she returned, we talked about her routine. "I just wish I could go one day," she confided, "without having to think about blood sugar levels, how much food I've had, what kind of food I will have, and by what time I need to have dinner." We looked at the people around us eating so many wonderful things in cream sauces and decided nobody in the room was thinking about diet and risk factors while they discussed stock options or the third race at Laurel. Both of us had been those people once. I told her, "I guess we could sit around and say 'Aw shucks,' but we have to move past that point eventually." She agreed.

The next time I was at that restaurant, I ordered a steak, well done. Just like the old times. But later in the day, I stayed on the treadmill 20 minutes longer to make up for my wayward afternoon. Today, if a steak at the Palm seems to have my name on it, I'm in the gym for an extra half hour to atone for my sins. Some will call that "excessive." I call it "the way things are." It works for me.

In 1997, I was thinking about "the way things could be." I had asked Shawn Southwick to be my wife and she agreed. We made plans for a spectacular wedding on a September evening in a Beverly Hills garden with Wolfgang Puck catering for 150 guests. I kept thinking how a poor Jewish kid from Brooklyn could never have dreamed of something so extravagant. The day before the ceremony, I went to the UCLA Medical Center to take what had become a routine stress test. I will admit I'd been feeling a little worn out, but I'd written it off as pressure to make the upcoming nuptials as wonderful as possible, while putting in some very long hours as a result of the sudden death of Princess Diana just a few days earlier. Shawn and I had plans for a romantic few weeks in Europe, and I wanted to have a doctor's word that my former heart troubles weren't going to reappear while walking with my beautiful bride past the shops in Paris.

Guess what?

I had another positive stress test (the adjective still doesn't make sense to me). The doctors were whispering quietly among themselves and throwing nervous glances my way until I was finally told that one of my arteries was going to have to be opened with angioplasty. And it was going to have to be done very soon. I said out loud, "Oh, son of a bitch!" I called Dr. Isom, and arrangements were made for me to fly to New York within the next 24 hours, have the procedure done there, and then spend a few days recuperating in a hospital room and a New York hotel instead of . . . well, need I even complete the sentence?

In place of a wedding on a Friday evening as the sun set across a beautiful garden, Shawn and I were married early in the morning in my hospital room. Yes, I thought about the dinner conversation—about wishing to have one day without dealing with a disease. But that's the way things are. Heart disease is something you don't just deal with once and it stays static. Subconsciously, you are dealing with it every single moment because things are changing all the time, and with each passing "now," you carry "the way things are" along. Yeah, it's frustrating. Don't I know. . . .

My work is one of the things that have pulled me through moments like this. It's a way of participating and being productive. But "work" can also mean a lot of other things besides what you do for a living. Maybe you can make the best turkey salad with oil and vinegar for lunch—that's still being "productive." Yet, there's also something that comes from inside, where no job description or recipe exists. I became that kind of "productive" while sitting in bed a few days after surgery, trying to concentrate on the pages of USA Today spread out in front of me detailing a mayoral election in Chicago and U.S. conflicts with the Duarte regime in El Salvador. I was unable to focus on news. Couldn't focus on baseball. Couldn't watch people whine on Oprah. This went on for a while because something was banging in my head saying, "Look at what's in front of you." I'm not talking about a bright light flashing in the sky and a chorus of harps playing from the clouds. It was more like the hand-drawn light bulb that you always see in the comic pages when someone suddenly hits on a new idea. I looked away from the news of the day and understood that there was another way I could be productive. I could see it. Yeah, right in front of me. And in deference to attention spans, it's a short story.

When I was a kid, my dad had a heart attack and died. It was sudden. Our family no longer had a paycheck coming in from his job building ships in a defense plant in Brooklyn. My mother was faced with supporting two kids, paying the rent, putting food on the table, and providing clothes for school. This was the same moment when I needed glasses, and there just wasn't any possible way we could afford them. Welfare covered the cost. New York allowed me the chance to see clearly for the first time in my life.

So sitting in that hospital room, I knew I was making very good money and the surgery and doctor's bills were covered 100 percent by insurance. But how, I wondered, can anyone afford this if they don't have medical coverage? Even though I couldn't concentrate on news or television talk shows, I was well aware of the fact that, at the time, 35 million people had no health insurance. (I knew this because I had done a radio show about it before you-know-what happened earlier in the year.) Today, that number is closer to 43 million people—more than 15 percent of the population. While presidents from both political parties have made attempts to improve how many people are covered, the only point on which there is agreement is that there is a long way to go . . . which isn't an answer at all. We are good at fixing health problems, but we are lousy at delivering an affordable way to have them fixed.

By the time I walked out of New York Hospital, I had a plan to find a way that would provide this life-saving surgery for working men and women and their children who are, through no fault of their own, without the financial resources to pay its cost. For whatever reason, they had fallen through the cracks in our health care system. Instead of doing one more interview about it, I decided to just *do* something about it. Today, the Larry King Cardiac Foundation is in its 15th year of providing funds for heart patients in need of life-saving surgery. Proceeds from this book will cover the cost of operations for people who, like that family in Brooklyn so many years ago, just can't afford to pay for something that's desperately needed in order to remain productive, or at least give them the chance to be so.

With heart disease, it's not just the body that heals—the mind does, too. And when both are able, get ready for one hell of a ride. These people and these pages are proof of where you can go.

To contact The Larry King Cardiac Foundation, log on to www.lkcf.org, or write to:

The Larry King Cardiac Foundation
15720 Crabbs Branch Way
Suite D
Rockville, MD 20855

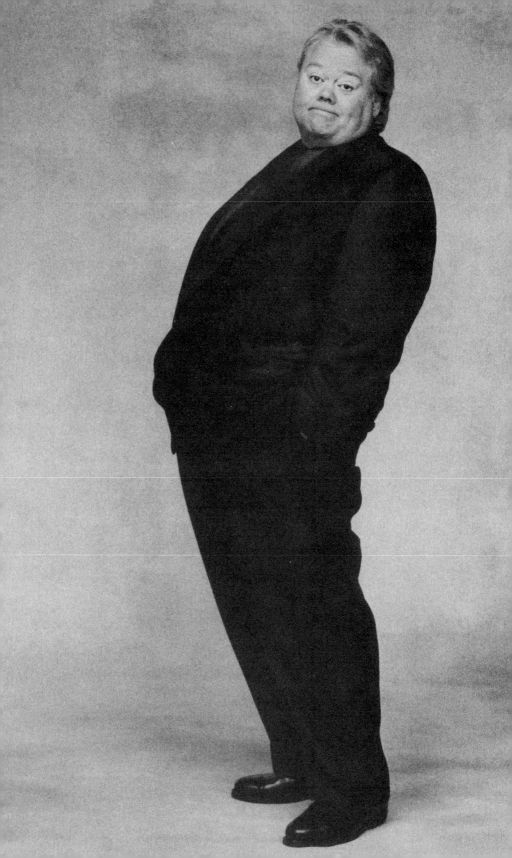

LOUIE ANDERSON

America first got to know Louie Anderson when the young comic from Minnesota appeared on The Tonight Show *with Johnny Carson. Long before anyone had heard the word "dysfunctional," Louie entertained audiences with jokes about the family. He went on to play every major comedy club in the country and hosted* Family Feud *for 3 years. The winner of two Emmys for his animated children's series* Life with Louie, *he has also written a number of best-selling books, including* Dear Dad: Letters from an Adult Child. *In September 2003, Louie was preparing to go back on the road when he made a turn into Cedars-Sinai Hospital.*

"It's not the end of the world and the end of your life because you have bypass surgery. I think people have to realize it's an opportunity to have a second look at what they're doing."

I see the scar on my chest every day, and it reminds me of the body's amazing ability to heal. While I was recovering from bypass surgery in the fall of 2003, I had moments when I asked myself, "What now? Am I going to have more health problems from now onward? Or is this the beginning of changing my life?" Now that some time has passed, I can see that the experience has changed me—and for the most part, it's been for the better.

The first time after the surgery when I was able to say, "I'm okay" was when I went back to work. It was November in Pittsburgh, and I was playing the Improv. There's a lot of moving around when you're onstage, and I was worried that I wouldn't be able to make it through a whole show. But as soon as I got onstage, I went right back into what I do. It all came back very naturally. I did 15 minutes on the experience with my heart. I talked about the fact that no matter how sick you are, if you're in a doctor's office or a hospital room, you still look around for stuff to steal. I remember looking through the drawers in my hospital room to see if there was anything I needed. You can never have enough gauze!

It all began in late September 2003. I was getting ready to go to Atlantic City to work at the Borgata and I was feeling okay, but not great. I guess I could best describe it as having low energy. I got up to get ready and I started having a discomfort in my chest. It wasn't a feeling I had known before—and it certainly wasn't a Taco Bell dysfunction. (See, if you're a food person like I am, you know your eating problems. This wasn't about that.) And my left arm was hurting. I said, "This just isn't right."

I decided to drive myself to Cedars-Sinai Medical Center. I was worried that I could be having trouble with my heart. There had been heart problems in my family. My dad had a heart problem and had to take medicine for it, although he didn't die of it. My mom died of a massive heart attack after having a complete physical 3 days earlier. And one of my brothers has been treated for cardiomyopathy. I just didn't want to take any chances.

I walked into the ER and as soon as I mentioned the words "chest pains," I was taken right in and put on a heart monitor. They also drew blood and took an EKG. My blood pressure was very high, but fortunately, they found that I hadn't had a heart attack. But because of my symptoms, they wanted to keep me overnight.

The next day, a cardiologist performed some tests, including an angioplasty. I'm a big guy, and you're on a table the size of an ironing board—it was very uncomfortable. I watched the procedure on a monitor and tried to joke with the doctors, but they weren't laughing. This was a tough crowd because they had a different agenda than I did. They wanted to tell me what was wrong, but I wanted them to tell me everything was okay.

The doctors found two blocked arteries and decided to put a

stent in each one to open them. They put one in, but when they attempted the second one, there was a curve in my artery and the catheter wouldn't make the bend. The next day, they brought in the big guns to try it again, but they were still unsuccessful.

The next step was bypass surgery, but I resisted the idea at first. I had done a stupid thing and watched one of those TV shows where they show a bypass being performed. Never watch one of those shows when it's possible you might eventually be the patient. Three days later, though, after talking with my family, friends, and my manager, I agreed to the operation.

I think that my belief in a higher power got me through the surgery. I didn't cut deals. I don't pray for stuff for myself. I said, "Here's a great opportunity. You're in one of the best hospitals in the world. Your heart hasn't been damaged. You really can't be asking for anything." I prayed for help for the doctor. I truly believe that it's not the end of the world and the end of your life because you have bypass surgery. I think people have to realize it's an opportunity to have a second look at what they're doing.

When I woke up after the surgery, I was in Intensive Care. I had a breathing tube in me, and I could feel pain in my chest. I remember being conscious but not being able to open my eyes or move. I could hear people talking—they were saying that I had a double bypass and that I was having some problems with bleeding. I learned that's a risk for people who are overweight. They tend to have bleeding after this type of surgery.

The doctors ended up taking me back into the OR to stop the bleeding. When I woke up later, I could open my eyes. After about 12 hours, they took the breathing tube out, which was a huge relief.

Recovery is strange. Your body is in shock from what it has

been through, and you just want to sleep. But I learned that the doctors and nurses give you only a very short grace period to recover. They want you up and doing things. They were very insistent that I get out of bed and try walking. My legs felt weak, but I was able to walk to the doorway of the room and back again. Personally, I preferred the idea of more pain medication instead of more walking, but I do think there's a part of every human being that knows movement is the right thing.

I have this advice for anyone facing bypass surgery: Look at it the same way you'd look at getting new tires for your car. It's just as unsafe to live with clogged arteries as it is to drive with bald tires. Think of the surgery as a way to prevent bigger problems. My friends didn't let me weasel out of it. I think once you leave the hospital, it becomes 100 times more difficult to return to have it done. The experience inspired me to think I had an opportunity to be healthier than I ever had been. And I haven't let that feeling go.

These days, I eat very little of the stuff that I know is bad. I got to a point where I said, "You know, I've already had all the bad food any human needs to have." Now, one of my meals each day is a salad. Even before the surgery, I had started to turn things around by being on the Zone diet—but the damage had already been done. I had grown up in Minnesota eating a lot of heavy food; and when I was on the road, I would finish a show around midnight, which meant that the only thing available was fast food. I didn't think about it then, but now I do.

Plus, I've become more active. I've always had a gym in my house, but it's a new addition as far as I'm concerned. After the surgery, I finally found out where it was. I guess it's never too late to start.

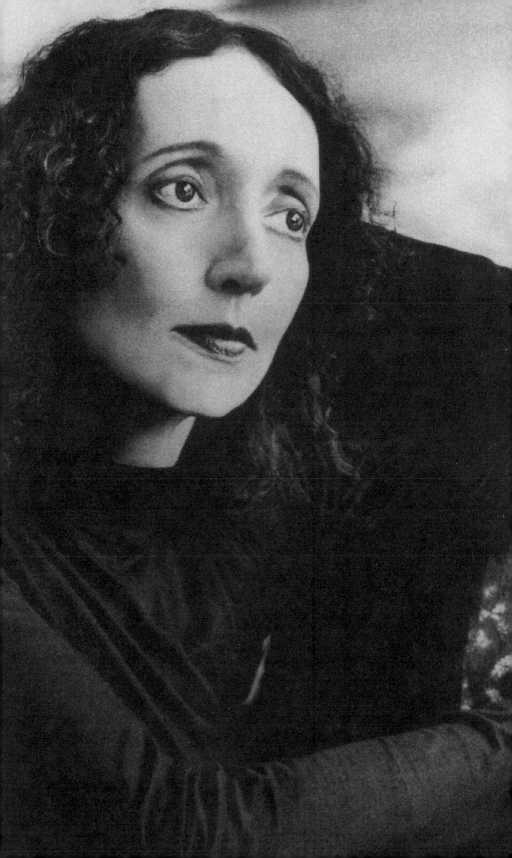

Joyce Carol Oates

A prolific writer at 65, Joyce Carol Oates is the Roger S. Berlind Distinguished Professor of Humanities at Princeton University. Since 1978, she has been a member of the American Academy of Arts and Letters. In 1970, she received the National Book Award for fiction; in 2003, the Common Wealth Award of Distinguished Service in Literature. Among her titles are the New York Times *bestseller* We Were the Mulvaneys, Black Water, *and* You Must Remember This. *Oates has lived her life with a condition called "mitral valve prolapse" (commonly known as a heart murmur), which can precipitate bouts of tachycardia (quickened heartbeat).*

"After so many years, it was important to finally get a diagnosis and have a name for the attacks I was experiencing."

I'm often chided for my productivity, but I do think there is a link between my heart condition and my reputation as a prolific writer. It's painful for me to knowingly waste time. I feel a sensation of acute unhappiness if I'm trapped in a situation in which I must waste time, and so I try to bring work materials or literature with me on trips and in waiting rooms, for instance. Since I write in longhand, on miscellaneous sheets and scraps of paper, I can write virtually anywhere.

Since the age of 18, I have suffered from tachycardia attacks, which can be fairly mild or quite severe. Basically, it is a quickened heartbeat. It is a "pounding," or "runaway," heartbeat. It's really quite astonishing, and if you experience such an attack, your entire body will rock and vibrate with the maniacal pounding of your heart—as if an angry fist were inside your ribcage, pounding to be released. The worst attack I've ever suffered (so far) involved a heartbeat of 250 to 270 beats a minute; the average is said to be about 100 to 150 beats per minute. The worst attacks necessitate emergency room help immediately, while the others can be "waited out." (At least, that has been my procedure. I have to admit that if anyone in my family were suffering an even average attack, I would probably insist upon taking him or her to the ER.)

During the attack, your thoughts are likely to be transcendent. Your body, or your brain, seems to believe that it is about to die, and so your thoughts are correspondingly ever more detached from your pounding heart. You think back over your life, you assess your life, you think of people whom you love, you think of the work you are doing that will not be completed—you are utterly helpless and so you give up resistance. This "giving up" is like relaxing a fist, in fact. I would like to say that the "giving up" signals a release from the violent attack, but it has nothing to do with it, and an attack can continue for a long time after such a transcendent moment. However, when the attack ends—which happens as abruptly as it began—you will immediately be bathed in a sensation of relief. You will think, "My life has been given back to me. Now I must use it wisely." For hours afterward, you bask in a new kind of serenity. You are very happy! Like the one who, in Yeats's words, is blessed and can bless.

I've sometimes felt that critics who judge me harshly because I write "too much" in their eyes might not judge me so harshly if they understood that I live each day, in fact each minute, under what seems to me a spell of mortality. I focus my energies on my work, on what is most important to me in my work, on writing what I hope will outlive me, because I've had numerous terrifying occasions when it did not seem to me that I would survive to continue working, or to complete a project I cared deeply about.

Yet I haven't lived my entire life this way. In high school, I had always been an enthusiastic athlete. I was captain of a volleyball team, and I played on basketball and field hockey teams. And so growing up, I had no sense of physical limitations of any kind. Then it happened that, at the age of 18, during a basketball game in a physical education class at Syracuse University, I was struck very hard by a hefty guard, knocked to the hardwood floor, and suddenly overcome by what seemed to be, at the time, a heart attack.

I could not breathe, my heart was racing, I may have fainted. I remember, most vividly, the gym teacher staring down at me with such horror, going deathly white, and nearly fainting herself. This attack, which I did not know to be a tachycardia attack, lasted for about 20 minutes, and then, mysteriously, abated. By this time, my fingers and toes were icy cold and I was exhausted.

I was able to walk to the infirmary, where I was "examined" and told to rest for a while. I remember lying on a cot while there and reading, or trying to read, an assignment for my literature class. I remember being in a state of suspended terror, perspiring, still exhausted, but diligently underlining passages in Wordsworth's rhapsodic but somewhat protracted "Prelude." I recall noting how the word "heart" is evoked, in naively abstract terms, as a synonym for "sensibility." But the heart is far more than merely refined poetic sensibility; it is an unpredictable physical organ, which no poetry can define. I remember also being determined not to allow the attack to interfere with my studies or my life generally.

It will sound strange in retrospect, in an era in which everyone is so health-conscious, but I didn't tell my parents about my attack, and I didn't tell my college friends. I didn't want to seem "different" or in any way at a disadvantage. Perhaps in some obscure way,

I felt ashamed of such a weakness and wanted to believe that it would never happen again. (I was excused from basketball for the rest of the semester. I have never played the game again.)

For many of the following years, I seem to have been in a state of denial about my cardiac condition. I thought that each attack was special and would not be repeated. Usually, you have to lie down immediately when you are having an attack, but I do recall a siege in Madison, Wisconsin, when I was a graduate student in English in the fall of 1960. I suffered an attack on the ground floor of the graduate women's residence hall, near the mailboxes in the lobby, and had to make my way—to "walk"—upstairs to my room on the second floor, an effort that required about one hour of "walking" by inches, clinging to the wall. It was a late hour of the night, and I didn't call for help.

At Madison, I was finally sent to a doctor who ordered blood tests, but oddly, did not arrange for any cardiac tests. (The blood results were ultimately "lost.") There was no diagnosis of any kind. I remember the doctor telling me that such attacks are "idiopathic."

Sometime in the 1980s, in Princeton, New Jersey, when I suffered a really extreme tachycardia attack, my husband took me to the emergency room of the Princeton Medical Center, where I was treated with an IV solution—and given a diagnosis. Finally, I had a cardiologist who thoroughly tested me and explained my condition. On a piece of paper he wrote these words, which I keep in a drawer:

Paroxysmal atrial tachycardia
Good amounts of exercise
Discontinue caffeine

LIVING LIFE WITH TACHYCARDIA

Raymond Smith and Joyce Carol Oates were married in January 1961. Since that time, Raymond has been present when Joyce has experienced a number of tachycardia attacks.

Joyce first told me about her "attacks" a few months before we were married. For years, I did not witness any of them. It is possible that Joyce hid them from me since she has never liked to dwell upon health matters. (This is an Oates family trait. The Oateses are good-natured stoics, or try to be.)

I have since learned that the severity of the attack dictates whether you must take the afflicted person to the ER immediately. I trust Joyce to tell me if she needs to go to the emergency room. I know that she will not exaggerate her condition but also will not allow it to become dangerous. I can never see an attack coming on, so I rely on her to tell me when she's experiencing symptoms.

It's important to listen to your cardiologist's advice and to follow the preventive measures he recommends. Joyce has always been quite athletic and runs every day and exercises in other ways, and perhaps this has helped her. But she would exercise in any case since she is a rather restless person when not deeply immersed in her work, which is the center of her imaginative life.

After so many years, it was important to finally get a diagnosis and have a name for the attacks I was experiencing. I used to drink tea with caffeine but have stopped entirely, of course, since I learned that there's a link between the attacks and stimulants like caffeine. I also don't drink anything with alcohol in it, and I don't smoke, nor did I preceding the tachycardia.

I've been prescribed to take one small white Lanoxin tablet every day, and I've had very few attacks over the past 20 years. Like other people suffering from this condition, I can feel an "attack" coming on and have learned to forestall it by instinctively holding my breath, or readjusting my body, or lifting my arms high above my head and stretching. Also, like most people suffering from this condition, I am acutely aware of how suddenly an attack can strike, at any time, at any place, in even the most relaxed of environments, like sleep.

Interestingly, I've never had an attack while giving a public reading or talk. When I'm being introduced on stage, my heartbeat doesn't even quicken. Personal public appearances don't make me at all nervous, and I do enjoy them. I have very little anticipation of any public event and absolutely no apprehension. In my case, at least, the tachycardia attacks are, indeed, "idiopathic" and not related to any sort of stress.

From childhood onward, I have been physically active, and I continue to be so today. The great love of my life is running. It's an understatement to say that I love running: I seem to require it for intellectual as well as physical reasons. Running daily, sometimes twice daily, is my "meditation" which helps immeasurably with my work. Dancing—nothing so stately as ballroom, but rather more the rhythmically strenuous/joyous motions of, for instance, a contemporary dance troupe like the Alvin Ailey—is equally wonderful.

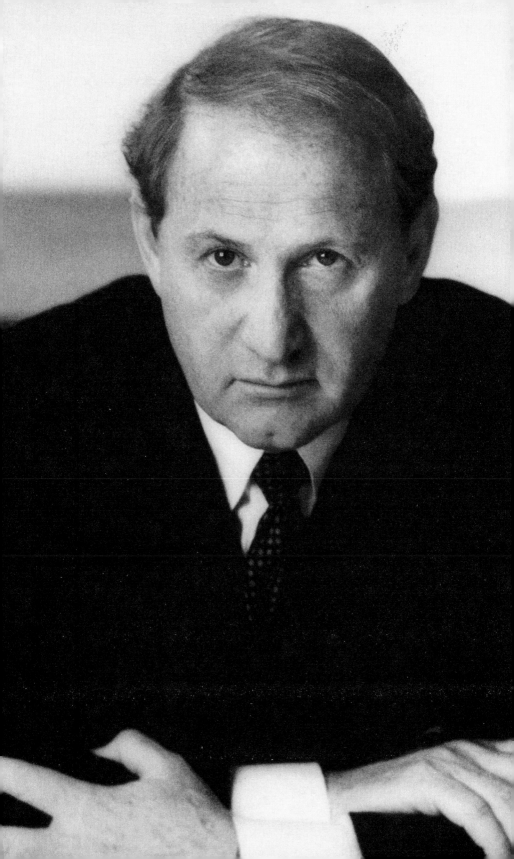

MIKE MEDAVOY

Mike Medavoy started off in the mailroom at Universal Pictures back in 1964. Since that time, he has accumulated seven Best Picture Oscars and become one of the country's top movie moguls. He produced Philadelphia, Bull Durham, Basic Instinct, Hannah and Her Sisters, *and* The Silence of the Lambs, *to name a few of his works. Today, the 62-year-old is head of Phoenix Pictures. He underwent surgery to repair a heart valve in 1999, and almost a year ago, he had a pacemaker implanted. He isn't one to look back, though—probably because he's always looking ahead to the next project.*

"I think that having a focus beyond your illness helps you to stay motivated throughout your recovery."

I'm not surprised by any of the heart problems I've had. Even though heart trouble doesn't run in my family, I think medical scares like the ones I've had are all a part of life. Life is full of surprises, and it's how you deal with them that matters. You just have to do your best and use what you've learned to try to figure out what life is all about. In my case, I've figured out what works for me. I have a different perspective on life now than I did 20 years ago.

I'm looking at the big picture now. As you get older, no matter whether you're sick or not, you look at your life differently. Everybody does, and if they don't, they're missing something important. I'm much more in tune with things that I didn't quite understand before. As I get older, I'm much wiser. I think this wisdom is related to my spiritual needs, an understanding of what my life was really like. You get distance from things and you get perspective—what you did right, what you did wrong. It's a matter of getting older, not of having heart surgery.

I think my heart problem started when I took fen-phen in

1999 as a way to lose weight. Prior to that, I hadn't had any heart problems. But pretty soon, I couldn't even walk up a flight of stairs. I felt like my body was shutting down. I also started having episodes of arrhythmia. It was my irregular heartbeat that started to worry me, so I finally went to see my doctor. This all took place 6 months before I ended up having surgery.

I wasn't in denial, but I sure didn't move toward a doctor very fast either. I guess I've always believed that when it comes to health issues, I'll get better even if I don't do anything. I wouldn't have gotten anything done if I hadn't been pressed. I feel like a lot of people do: I can self-medicate and take care of it without seeing a doctor. So it wasn't until I reached a point where I really wasn't feeling well that I finally went ahead and got a series of x-rays and stuff like that. I then went to a doctor who told me, "You know, I think the valve is going to have to be repaired. You have to take care of it."

I immediately said, "I want a second opinion and I want to go to somebody who's the world expert on this. Give me a name." He gave me the name of a doctor in San Francisco, so I flew up there and met with him. After evaluating me, that doctor said, "I don't think you need it . . . yet." So I returned to Los Angeles and said, "I don't need it." That was what I wanted to hear, and so I decided to go with it. I decided I didn't need to do a thing.

Still, I could feel my heart going in and out of rhythm. It happened anywhere. There wasn't any specific moment or activity when I would feel it, so I never knew when to expect it. I didn't get tired. I didn't feel well, but I never had any pain. I would just get out of breath, though it was never very bad. But I was told that it was getting to be dangerous to allow my heart to go in and out of rhythm as it was doing, and so I finally agreed to surgery to repair my heart valve. Looking back, I think I probably had to be talked into it. The surgery was scheduled to be done at the UCLA Medical Center.

Throughout the days leading up to the heart valve surgery, I was pretty much at peace with my decision. I think it's important for anyone facing heart surgery to have confidence in their decision and in their doctors. I wasn't worried about anything. This is not a town where you can keep a secret, and, quite frankly, I don't know that anyone other than your friends cares. On the night before the surgery, the doctor came into my hospital room and we talked about my other interests. I discovered that we both have an interest in history, and that was a good way to keep from thinking about what would happen in the hours to come.

After the operation, Arnold Schwarzenegger called me from Europe to ask if I was okay. In fact, his was the first phone call I got after the operation. In the months before the surgery, I was producing *The 6th Day*, and Arnold and I had talked a little about the surgery I was about to undergo. We had a nice talk that day. He had a valve replacement. I just had a repair. I think it's helpful to talk with someone who's been through a similar experience and to look to their recovery for motivation for your own.

Soon, though, I learned that the operation had solved only part of the problem. My heart was still going in and out of rhythm. I was told I needed a pacemaker, but I fought it. I couldn't actually feel the arrhythmia any longer, so I wasn't troubled by it. I could still do whatever I wanted to do. I could even play tennis. But one day, I had a scare that sent me to the hospital; the doctors thought it might have been a minor stroke. And so I finally agreed that it was time to address the problem. In June 2003, I had a pacemaker implanted, but now only half of it is working; the bottom half works but the top half doesn't. My heart had some scarring as a result of the operation to repair the heart valve problem, so it was difficult for the doctors to connect the pacemaker. It just means my heart operates at 10 percent less efficiency than a normal heart. I do go back to the cardiologist from time to time and have a pacemaker interrogation done, and everything seems to be okay—despite the fact that I am missing 10 percent efficiency.

Everyone has their own unique issues they must deal with when faced with heart surgery and the recovery process. For me, and for others like me who are used to dealing with powerful people, heart disease seemed like a personal attack. It's easy for us to talk ourselves out of going through with the surgery. But it's not a personal attack, and it's not something you can talk yourself out of.

When you're doing well in life, you want to believe you're controlling everything, including your own life. But having a medical problem teaches you that control is only in your mind. Yet this discovery ultimately helps you to look more deeply at your life. I've always been somebody who has searched for answers. I've never just accepted every answer that came along. I was somebody who had some sort of philosophical sense of my life. And as you get older, and especially as you start to face issues with your health, you get more philosophical and you start to find out more and more about what surrounds you.

Moving On with My Responsibilities

Since the pacemaker was implanted, there have been some times when I've felt more depressed than I should, and I have no idea what that's about. I've also found myself becoming much more pensive. I've always been fairly even-keeled emotionally, at least on my exterior, so this has been a new experience for me. It has never gotten in the way of anything I've tried to do, though. I'm able to be at peace with the whole thing.

In the autumn of 2003, I had a seizure. I got up and went to the bathroom and my wife came in and I guess I must have passed out or something. There are pieces of my memory that are erased. She called 9-1-1, and I woke up on the way to the hospital in an ambulance. All the tests showed everything was normal, but now I'm on medication for seizures. My medical conditions have kind of compounded themselves one on top of the other. I try to moderate the things I do in terms of not getting involved in as much as I used to. Having said that, though, I'm currently working on a book about movies over the past 100 years that have had an impact on leadership. Plus, I'm on the board of the Kennedy School of Government at Harvard, I'm involved in the California governor's anti-terrorist organization, and I'm still doing movies.

As to what got me through this, well, I've gotten through a lot of things in my life. My wife has been an unbelievable supporter, and she has been there for me when I've needed her. She's propped me up, even though I'm usually the type of guy who says, "Okay, I don't need any propping." But you know, I think a lot of it has to do with the fact that I didn't let myself worry

TAKE HEART

- *It's normal to feel anxious or fearful after being diagnosed with a heart problem or undergoing cardiac surgery. Finding a number of people that you can confide in—such as your spouse, close friends, or a counselor—will help you to feel stronger mentally and put you on the path to recovery.*
- *Remember that you are not alone: There are more people than ever before who are leading full and active lives after heart surgery. Concentrating on a goal or event that you can look forward to will help you to gain a perspective outside of your illness.*

about it too much. I have a 5½-year-old child and a 38-year-old and my parents are still alive, so I have a lot of responsibility, and I'm trying to make sure that all of it gets taken care of. I think that having a focus beyond your illness helps you to stay motivated throughout your recovery.

I think I've had a good attitude going through this. I never thought, "This ain't gonna work." And I never felt sorry for myself. I never did the "Why me?" thing. I'm not scared that my heart could act up again. My advice to other people facing heart surgery is that before you have it, make peace with yourself. I did that prior to the surgery. I've made a lot of mistakes. But I tell myself that whatever it is, and whatever is coming, is coming. What I'm here to do now is to make a better life for others. Being friends with yourself is the most important thing. I'd like to hang around for my kids and for my wife. In the end, I know I'm doing okay.

On the Trail of a Deadly Diet Drug

Sometimes, doctors also have to be detectives. The first person to suspect that the once popular diet drug fen-phen (fenfluramine-phentermine) might cause heart valve problems was Dr. Hartzell Schaff, an expert in heart valve repair at the Mayo Clinic. In May 1996, a patient with a damaged mitral valve was referred to Dr. Schaff.

During surgery, Dr. Schaff noted the unusual appearance of the valve: It was thickened, with a glistening white exterior. It reminded him of the way valves look that have been damaged by medications used for migraines, such as ergotamine. But the patient had no history of taking ergotamine, and an echocardiogram taken 2 years earlier revealed no abnormalities. After the surgery, Dr. Schaff spoke with the patient, who said that she hadn't taken any migraine medicines, but she had taken fen-phen for 25 months prior to surgery. He went to the pharmacy at Mayo and asked whether heart problems had ever been reported with this combination of medications. No connection had ever been made, but Dr. Schaff remained suspicious.

The patient recuperated from surgery and was discharged, but a week later she developed leg swelling and shortness of breath. Dr. Schaff ordered another echocardiogram, which revealed that the repaired mitral valve was fine, but the tricuspid valve on the other side of the heart was leaking severely. Dr. Schaff asked me to take a look at the patient and the echocardiogram. When I saw her, I too became suspicious when she talked about her use of fen-phen. I researched how these medications work to decrease appetite and discussed the drugs and their effects with several nutrition specialists. We strongly suspected that the diet drugs had caused valve disease in this patient. This was a concern since they were very popular (the total number of monthly prescriptions for fen-phen exceeded 18 million in 1996).

Working with several individuals from the Mayo Clinic as well as MeritCare in Fargo, North Dakota, we identified 24 women who had had no prior history of cardiac disease but, after using fen-phen, developed symptoms of a heart murmur or other cardiovascular trouble. Of these patients, three required valve replacement surgery. The valve tissue pathology from these patients helped us to confirm the link we suspected.

Our findings were released to the FDA and the public in July 1997 and published the next month in the *New England Journal of Medicine*. In between those times, the FDA arranged for testing and found there was a much higher frequency of valve disease in people who had used fen-phen (30 percent) than the frequency expected in the regular population (5 to 6 percent). At the government's urging, the pharmaceutical company elected to withdraw fenfluramine and dexfenfluramine from the market in September 1997.

It should be noted that more women than men were affected by fen-phen because many more women than men took these diet drugs. However, both men and women are vulnerable to the drugs' damaging effects, and men who took the drugs were affected just as frequently as women who took them.

—HEIDI CONNOLLY, M.D., *associate professor of medicine at Mayo Medical School in Rochester, Minnesota, and consultant on cardiovascular diseases*

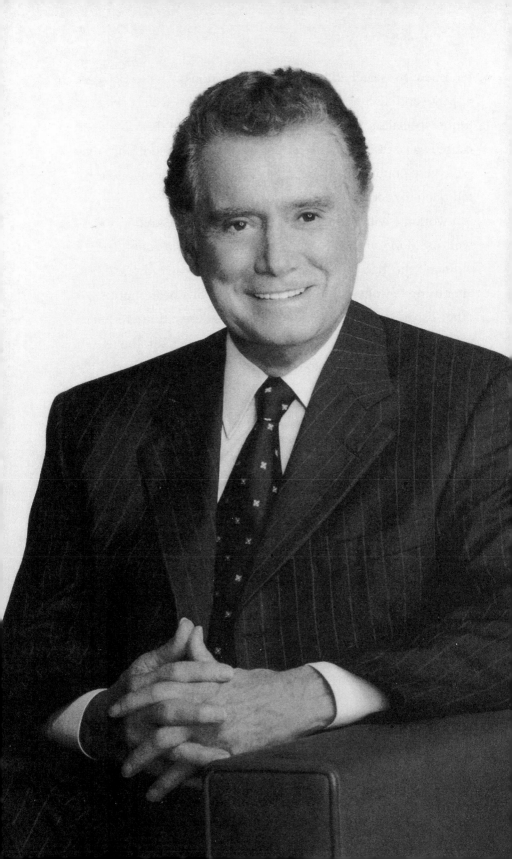

REGIS PHILBIN

Regis was the sidekick on The Joey Bishop Show *from 1967 to 1969. Twenty years later, he was paired with Kathie Lee Gifford for one of the most popular morning television talkfests in history, which continues to this day with co-host Kelly Ripa. Regis began working two jobs in 1999, when he was named host of the game show* Who Wants to Be a Millionaire, *which has delivered great ratings. He is 78 years old and talks about slowing down. It still hasn't happened.*

"I had been lifting weights since I was a teenager in the Bronx, but I hadn't exercised the most important muscle in my body: my heart."

One day in 1991, I was scheduled to do a television commercial for Carnival Cruise Line with my co-host at the time, Kathie Lee Gifford. I had done two TV shows that morning. My flight to the Caribbean was an hour late taking off, and I missed a connecting flight to the island where the ship was docked. The trip had already been very stressful, and I hadn't even reached the ship. Finally, I got there via helicopter, which landed about 500 yards from the ship at dock. I carried two heavy bags of luggage to the gangplank. Needless to say, by the time I got to my room, I was exhausted.

That night, I felt a pounding in my chest. I thought it would pass. It didn't. I called sick bay and arranged to meet the ship's doctor. He took an electrocardiogram, which showed nothing. Still, the pain persisted and the doctor advised me to go to Mount Sinai Hospital in Miami Beach when the ship docked later that day and have a more thorough checkup before flying home to New York City. I almost took a pass, but decided at the last minute to go through with it. The pain had subsided and, I thought, so had the danger.

The personnel at Mount Sinai had been alerted to my situation by the ship's doctor. A few minutes after arriving, I was on a gurney being pushed into an operating room for an angiogram. They had sedated me slightly and had run a catheter from my groin into the heart area. I remember looking at the overhead monitors and marveling over seeing the inside of my heart. Suddenly, I felt very vulnerable. I tried to reassure myself by thinking that maybe they would find nothing wrong. The doctor gave me a running commentary as the search continued, and finally they found one artery that was 90 percent blocked. I could actually see the blockage on the monitor.

The doctor asked me if I would like him to proceed with an angioplasty because he could do it right there. It would take 45 minutes. How could I say no? And that's how it happened. My angioplasty was a wake-up call. I had been lifting weights since I was a teenager in the Bronx, but I hadn't exercised the most important muscle in my body: my heart.

Yes, I had eaten too much steak, too much ice cream, and too many eggs. And I hadn't done the cardiac work I should have. I never got involved in the jogging craze. Hated running. Didn't like the treadmill. I never really thought that heart disease could happen to me. And the news came as a big surprise to my wife, Joy. I didn't have a chance to tell her that I was going to the hospital. At least there was a happy ending when I did call.

I still hate to run, so I walk fast on an outdoor track at the Reebok Sports Center on Columbus Avenue in New York City, weather permitting. I work out on a treadmill in the winter. And I now eat more chicken and fish and less red meat. I'm not a saint about it, but I am more aware of my diet than I was

A REVOLUTIONARY TEST FOR DETECTING HEART DISEASE

Before long, emergency room doctors will have a new blood test to better predict whether a patient who is experiencing chest pain is on the brink of having a heart attack. Current tests, such as troponin blood tests and electrocardiograms (EKGs), are limited in that they often don't detect heart attacks until hours after they've occurred—and after the heart muscle has already been damaged. The new test will measure the level of an enzyme called myeloperoxidase (MPO) in the bloodstream. An elevated MPO level signals that the patient is at risk for an imminent heart attack. This test also has increased the ability to identify which patients are at future risk for a major cardiac event over the next 30 days to 6 months. In the past, tests could predict future risks 50 percent of the time, but the MPO test is able to predict the risk of a heart attack 85 to 95 percent of the time.

The MPO test is a simple blood test, which in one form will be administered with a special hand-held device, providing results faster, right at the patient's bedside. An elevated MPO level

before. And I'm more aware of my heart than ever before.

Incidentally, the doctor who performed the angioplasty told me there was a 40 percent chance that my artery might clog up again within 6 weeks. One afternoon as I filmed a segment with Cirque du Soleil, I felt a familiar pain in my chest. I finished the stunt and told my producer, Michael Gelman, what was hapin people with cardiovascular disease indicates arterial inflammation. Previous studies have linked this type of inflammation to increased risk of cardiovascular events.

A study of 604 emergency room patients by a team at the Cleveland Clinic sought to determine whether MPO was also a predictor of vulnerable plaque. Such fatty deposits in the arteries can become fragile and break off, cutting off blood flow to vital organs, such as the heart or brain, thereby causing heart attack or stroke. Other ways to measure arterial inflammation, such as the C-reactive protein (CRP) tests, also help doctors to gauge the risk of cardiac events. But in head-to-head comparisons in the emergency room setting, CRP testing was much less effective than MPO testing.

In addition to its use in the ER, scientists predict that in the future, the MPO test will become a common procedure offered in doctors' offices. By helping to identify those people who have heart disease but don't know it, the test could save thousands of lives each year.

—STANLEY HAZEN, M.D., *section head of preventive cardiology at the Cleveland Clinic Foundation*

pening, and he drove me to New York Presbyterian Hospital. Sure enough, the blockage was back. This time, I underwent an atherectomy (this procedure uses a rotating laser catheter that "shaves" the plaque off an artery). Thankfully, the pain has never returned. The artery remains open and functioning, and I couldn't be happier about it.

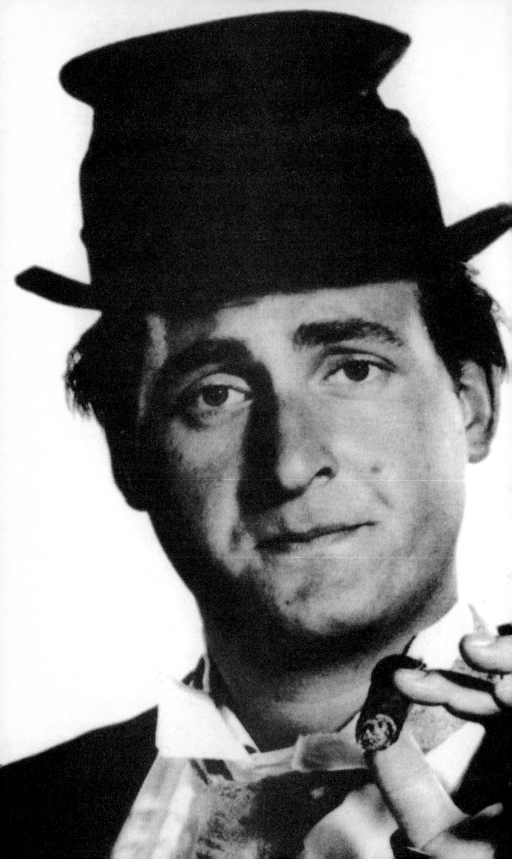

SID CAESAR

Sid is a television pioneer. He hosted Your Show of Shows *from 1950 to 1954, which teamed him with Imogene Coca for some of the greatest comedy routines ever aired. In 1963, he was in* It's a Mad, Mad, Mad, Mad World, *and today, at age 82, Sid Caesar has recovered from heart arrhythmia and bypass surgery.*

"I don't get mad like I used to before I had heart surgery. . . . Today, I treasure every moment and try not to waste it on things that don't mean anything."

I keep myself under control. I don't get mad like I used to before I had heart surgery. Look, if a guy cuts you off, you have to say to yourself, "I'm never going to see him again in my life. Never, ever. So am I going to risk my life and my family and everything I've worked for because of that?" No, no, no. Let him go. Enjoy your life. That's really the most important thing. And I'm talking about doing that every day.

Today, I treasure every moment and try not to waste it on things that don't mean anything. Something that happened yesterday is a "was." If it happens right now, then it's a "here." Don't waste time with the "was," and don't worry about the "gonna be." Spend your time with the "here"—that's how you move on with your life, and that's how you enjoy it.

When things started going wrong in 1985, I could tell pretty quickly. I could tell my heart was beating faster than normal. You feel it, especially when you lie down. Now, I have no idea where I was, but I knew something wasn't right. And I will tell you I was very afraid. I went to the doctor right away, and after he did some tests and listened to my heart, he told me I had an arrhythmia. He prescribed quinidine and digitalis. He also told me to lay off caffeine and chocolate, which I did.

After the diagnosis, I had to learn that getting excited about it wasn't going to help anything. You have to sit back and try to get yourself to calm down. You have to say, "Enough." I mean that. You gotta just say the hell with it. It ain't worth it. So I made an effort not to get wound up all the time. And you know what? Right away I was able to do that. I would say, "What the hell should I worry for?" I decided that I wanted to hang around and see how this all turns out.

I did what my doctor told me to do, at least for the most part. I tried to watch my diet, but I wasn't very serious about it. And 8 years later, my cardiologist said that I needed a bypass. He told me my body had made its own bypass around the blocked artery by using the surrounding small blood vessels, and that was probably a benefit of the 2-hour workouts I did every day. But now, he told me that my body couldn't handle it anymore, and it was time for bypass surgery. That hit me. It was a wake-up call. Having the arrhythmia got me thinking, but my doctor later said my whole attitude changed as soon as it was clear I was going to need a bypass.

When I was facing bypass surgery, I never thought about death. You can't think that way. If you do, if you think it isn't going to work or you aren't going to live, then why have the operation? Why spend the money? If you think like that, then the hell with it. You have to trust the doctor. He's the expert. He knows more than you know about a heart. If the doctor tells you "you gotta have surgery," then you gotta have it.

You have to make up your mind about what it takes to live. Either you want to keep taking the nitroglycerin pills or you decide that surgery is something that has to be done. Find the best surgeon you can. He isn't going to find you. You have to really know the person. Do research. Know the team, because all heart surgeons work as a team. That's what I did. I asked friends I knew who have heart disease. I got advice from doctors I knew. I kept saying to everyone I asked, "Look, this is my heart, so I have to know who is going to touch it."

You may go through a period of fear and worry about what's going to happen. Well, this is the main office, you know? And if the surgeons do a good job, this can mean additional years and years and years. I know.

On the night before my bypass, I was making all sorts of deals with God. This was a big operation—I wasn't going in to get a tooth pulled, after all. So I just hoped that everything would go all right. Everybody is different, and who knows? It was like a movie. I remember thinking to myself, "Okay, this is it." They put you under and that's it. When you come out . . . oh, it's marvelous. It's a whole new life.

I looked at surgery this way: If you know it's going to be bad and you keep saying you don't want to go, then you're defeating yourself. If you don't want to go, then don't go. That will be the end of it. But if you do go, you have to focus on the good that you hope to get out of the surgery. You need to concentrate on becoming healthy again and feeling better. If you fight the surgery, you're fighting against yourself.

Everybody who visited while I was in the hospital made me feel better. Boy, oh boy. That's when it means something to you—not that a visit doesn't always mean something. I was in the hospital for 6 days after the bypass. Dr. Cannom told me my recovery was "on target and uncomplicated." I did what had to be done, and I did it with a new view. I realized that I have a role in all of this.

Taking Small Steps to a Full Recovery

It took me 2 to 3 months before I started feeling good again. My advice is to give yourself time and try not to rush your recovery. And while you're doing that, exercise a little bit every day . . . just a little bit. Like get up and walk across the room. Start with that. That's wonderful. If you can do that two or three times a day, you're on your way. You have to learn how to walk, and then you have to learn how to live, and then, well, let live.

Since the bypass, I've gotten more serious about my diet. I eat the same thing each day: Every morning I eat tuna fish or salmon with a little olive oil, garlic, basil, oregano, and some nonfat yogurt (no mayonnaise). Yes, I eat that in the morning. And I walk. I used to work out for 2 hours every day, but I can't do that anymore. Now I walk through the hills in the morning, and that takes from 45 minutes to an hour.

I worked a little bit after the bypass surgery, but I started to

TAKE HEART

- *Recovering from heart surgery requires patience, but setting short-term goals for yourself can keep you motivated. Starting with a short walk, and then adding distance as you feel stronger, will allow you to see your progress.*
- *Research has shown that anger and stress can contribute to heart disease. Yoga, visualization, and exercise can help you to feel calmer and deal with problems more effectively.*

question why I was doing it. Instead, I decided it was time to retire. Retirement is great: You don't have to be anywhere. You don't have to say something. You don't have to make anybody laugh. You don't have to do anything. You want to leave, leave. You want to take a walk? Take a walk.

Retirement has also changed my attitude. After I retired, I told my wife, "That's it, I don't want any arguments. You win." We don't argue about anything. I just throw up my hands and say, "Okay, you win." That's different from the way I used to do it. Today I don't worry about anything. I don't feel guilty about anything. That's a "was" and there's nothing I can do about that. It's gone. I do the "now."

But at the same time, my new attitude doesn't mean I've become complacent. If you don't learn, you can forget about being successful. A lot of us don't really take the time to learn. We'll say, "Oh sure, I know what you mean" or "Yeah, I'm with you on that." But a lot of times, we don't take the time or make the effort to *truly* understand. But when you stop and take the time to understand something, then you really know what it's all about. You learn by yourself. Every day is precious. Enjoy it. Don't waste it on being mad. You've got to allow yourself to forget some things. You've got to allow yourself to learn new things. You are in charge of you. You see what you want to see.

⌯

The Doctor's Notes:
PUTTING PATIENTS IN CONTROL
OF THEIR HEALTH

DAVID CANNOM, M.D., director of cardiology at Good Samaritan Hospital
in Los Angeles, managing partner of Los Angeles Cardiology Associates
(an 18-physician cardiology group specializing in coronary
and electrophysiology interventions), and clinical professor of medicine
at the UCLA School of Medicine

Sid Caesar is a Type A personality who, for most of his life, was stressed and angry. He was drinking and wasn't getting much exercise. In 1985, he developed arrhythmia, which was probably triggered by stress—and anger. (Arrhythmia can also be triggered by such things as a severe lack of sleep or the caffeine in coffee or chocolate.) When a person experiences one, all, or a combination of these, his or her body increases its production of adrenaline. If the person has a bad heart, the result can sometimes be fatal. In Sid's case, he had to learn to take control of how he reacts to things, and he has become the poster boy for doing just that.

I treated Norman Cousins for 10 years prior to his writing *The Healing Heart*, and we learned together how a patient can heal outside of using the latest technology. Laughter has always provided relief in medicine, but in these modern times, we aren't teaching alternative holistic approaches in medical schools as much as we should be. It is my hope that this will change in the future.

The patient needs two things from a doctor: a sense that he or she is being taken care of, and a direct line of communication with that doctor. We need a horizontal playing field in which the patient and doctor are at equal levels and talk to each other, rather than the vertical playing field where the patient is being talked down to. This means I have to spend time with my patients, many of whom come in with a list of questions they've taken from research on the Internet—but that's what they need to feel comfortable with me. And that's how I treated Sid. We communicated. We talked. I learned not just about his heart, but about him as well. This is important and, unfortunately, it's overlooked too often because our medical system doesn't allow for this approach. Instead, doctors have too many patients on their daily schedule and this type of conversation isn't taking place. The truth is that technology is making it more and more difficult to have time for a patient.

Still, I think the future of medicine is bright. The patient— and the doctor—has to know the doctor isn't in control of everything that is occurring inside the body. So if the patient can control certain things, such as anger and stress, that patient is going to do better. Sid has done just that, and his experience with heart surgery was a transforming event for him. The fact that he eats like a monk, walks every day, and puts a limit on his emotions makes me feel confident enough to say that he has a better chance of dying from a falling coconut than from a heart condition. ▧

Angiogenesis:
The Body's Natural "Bypass"

The human body's ability to heal itself has always astounded those who study it, but some people seem to have a natural defense against cardiac damage that is nothing short of amazing. Each of us has numerous, tiny blood vessels called *collateral blood vessels*. When plaque buildup begins to block an artery, the bodies of certain individuals will respond by slowly growing these collateral vessels to compensate for the lack of blood flowing through the narrowed artery. In some cases—and Sid Caesar is an example of this—the collaterals will create a natural bypass, known as an *angiogenesis*.

The process begins when the partially or fully blocked artery releases proteins into nearby tissues, which in turn will attach to the cells of nearby blood vessels. Over a period of time, new blood vessels, or collaterals, grow toward the blocked artery. Unfortunately, many people with atherosclerosis (also called hardening of the arteries) who don't see a doctor will die before the collaterals can bypass the clogged area of the artery. The fact that Sid began exercising and controlling his diet are factors in the growth of these collateral vessels. But that wasn't enough to avoid bypass surgery because his arteries had also developed high-grade lesions (a deterioration of the artery wall as a result of a buildup of plaque).

No one is sure why certain individuals, but not others, are able to form collaterals. Scientists are currently looking to gene therapy in the hope that it will provide a way that we might stimulate and develop the growth of new blood vessels in those people whose bodies don't naturally have this ability. In addition, future research may help us understand how the body is able to form increased collaterals. Once we understand that, I believe we'll move quickly to find a way for the body to use angiogenesis and, maybe one day, decrease the number of bypass operations we do.

> —DAVID CANNOM, M.D., *director of cardiology at Good Samaritan Hospital in Los Angeles, managing partner of Los Angeles Cardiology Associates, and clinical professor of medicine at the UCLA School of Medicine*

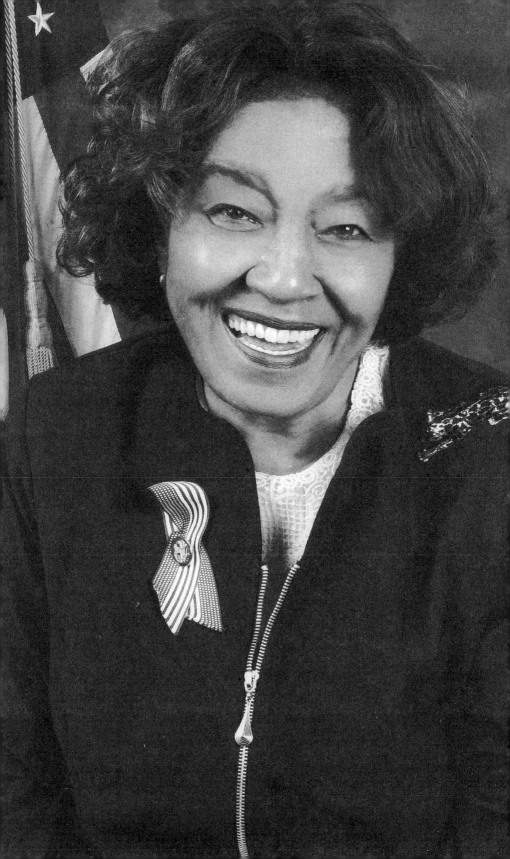

JULIA CARSON

Julia Carson served 18 years in the Indiana General Assembly as both a state representative and a senator from Indianapolis. In 1996, she was elected to Indiana's 10th Congressional District (as a result of redistricting, it is now the 7th) and became the state's first African-American member of Congress. It was a campaign that almost killed her, and politics wasn't the reason. At age 58, Julia Carson's heart was losing a battle with blocked arteries.

"Heart disease is a wake-up call that you need to change some things in your life. And when you do, you'll be stronger than ever."

I was running for Congress in 1996. Although I'm typically an energetic person, I started feeling tired all the time. I have always been an early morning person, getting up at 4 or 5 o'clock and letting it roll. But I could tell my steamboat was slowing down. I couldn't get it together like I was accustomed to doing. So I went to the doctor.

I had been on the Senate Health Committee in the Indiana General Assembly, and just from hearing people testify before our committee I knew about some of the health problems that can happen. I was feeling bad. I would get up and sit on the side of my bed and wouldn't feel like moving around. I didn't feel any pain at all. I was just without energy, and I had tingling in my hands and feet.

I went to my family physician and said, "Hey doc, I think this ol' ticker is getting ready to mess up and you need to check it out." He looked at me and said, "Mrs. Carson, there ain't nothing wrong with your heart." I said I wished that were true, but I was afraid that it wasn't. So I asked him again to run the tests so we could see what was up. Well, he kept insisting there wasn't anything wrong with my heart, and I kept arguing with him. I said, "You don't even know." Finally, he agreed to run a battery of tests, and when the nurse called, I went back to his office.

He told me I had high cholesterol, I was too fat, and I had high blood pressure, and I said, "I already know all of that." I knew I wasn't eating right. I ate a lot of fattening foods because that's my culture—collard greens, fatback, fried pork chops, and all that kind of stuff. And my mother was the best cook in the world. She could make lemon cakes and lasagna that would make you holler they were so good.

When the doctor got done looking at the results of the tests, he said, "By the way, we didn't look at your heart."

I got angry. I said, "If I were a man and came in here, you'd check my heart, wouldn't you?" We laughed about it, but in the back of my mind I knew this was my last visit with him. And I also knew I had a hell of a race to win, so I walked out his door feeling disgusted and still feeling awful.

I went back to campaigning, and it was a hard race, but I won. On January 3rd, I was busy wrapping up some things before I was due to leave for Washington a few days later to be sworn in as a U.S. Representative from Indiana's 10th District. That day, I was scheduled to see some people who were mad at me as a result of the just-completed campaign. I wanted to see if we could become friends again now that the election was past. But I was still feeling so tired.

I went to the meeting, but I remember I didn't want to sit down for fear I'd pass out. We spoke for a few minutes and I recall saying, "Okay, you all, I got to go now." I got back in my car and called my grandson's boss and said that I was driving over and that I needed my grandson to take me to the hospital. And then I called the hospital and said I was going to come in because I just wasn't feeling good at all and I thought I might be having a heart attack.

When I arrived at my grandson's workplace, he got in the car and drove me straight to the hospital. I was feeling really bad by this point. My grandson walked me into the emergency room, where I was met by the staff, who kept saying, "We've been looking for you." I later learned they had sent an ambulance and the fire department over to my house as a result of my earlier phone call, and when they couldn't get me to answer the door, they broke it down (and part of the front wall), did a search, and couldn't find me. I never once thought about calling 9-1-1. I really didn't want any of the drama that's always part of an ambulance ride. Yes, that was a bad judgment call, and I hope that others will learn from my experience and not hesitate to call an ambulance.

There were television and radio and print reporters in the ER. It turned out that a little old lady had run over somebody, and reporters from the local television stations were there to cover the story. But when I walked in, one of the nurses said, "Here she is!" and so the cameras started hanging around there.

The doctors examined me and ran tests, and that's about all I remember. I was feeling so tired. But I do recall one of them saying something about "clogged arteries." They brought in a cardiovascular surgeon named Dr. Daniel Beckman, who informed me that I needed emergency heart surgery. I remember saying, "Oh my goodness, I'm going to have to think about that." I mean, I was supposed to be in Washington in a few days to be sworn in.

Dr. Beckman told me, "You don't have time to think about it." I think that was, in a way, kind of good because you really *don't* have time to think about it. You just have to let it roll. Later, I learned he had told my family it looked bad. And then 5 days after the double bypass surgery I had a stroke, so they had to bring me back into the OR to take care of a blockage in my carotid artery. Two operations in just a few days. Little did I know.

A CAMPAIGN OF HEALING

I wasn't aware that people were afraid for me. I wasn't aware that my family and friends were gathered there in the hospital waiting room all night waiting to hear how I was doing. They were afraid of the outcome. But I didn't have time to get scared. When I first opened my eyes after the surgery, I remember seeing them and giving everyone a thumbs up. And one of my buddies was there. I gave him a signal as best I could that I was cold, and he ran and got a nurse to get me some blankets.

After the operation, I watched myself on TV because so many people thought I was "out of here." The local news stations had pulled out a lot of video clips about things I'd been doing as a community activist, and I watched it thinking it was like a memorial film of some kind.

I was so moved that every church in Indianapolis, Black and White, had me on their prayer list. I know that prayers helped me. Absolutely! God wasn't ready to take me on yet.

A federal judge in Indianapolis had a judge swear me in to Congress at the hospital. I asked Dr. Beckman to be a witness along with then-Governor Evan Bayh. I didn't even get to Washington for a couple of weeks, and then when I did get there, I still wasn't feeling well.

When I did get to Congress, it was a very tearful kind of experience. It was spiritual. I had thought about it for so long and worked so hard and then I had my heart problem—but I was here. One of the Congressional papers ran a headline saying "Julia Carson Reaches Congress . . . Finally."

As much as I wanted to be in Washington, after 3 days I ended up coming back home. I wanted to be near my doctors. They checked me out again and did a second procedure on my other carotid artery. This is where they go into your neck and scrape away plaque that has accumulated. (The carotid artery provides the main supply of blood to the brain from the aorta.) The doctors explained that this procedure would keep me from having another stroke, since a narrowed carotid artery is the primary cause of stroke. I thought about everything that lay ahead of me, but I was focused on getting well. I told the doctors, "Let's make a day of it, no matter how long it takes."

I was in the hospital for 2 days, and during that time, I understood from conversations with nurses that the time of post-surgery can be just as dangerous as the actual surgery. I wanted to feel good again because I wanted to do a good job in Washington. And it was only later that I thought about the fact I'd just gone through three operations within a month.

LESSONS LEARNED

I know that many people who are reading this book are facing heart disease, and for them I have some advice: First, be encouraged because medical science is so advanced now and there are more people than you can imagine who are walking around after bypass surgery. Second, remember that you are going to feel so much better after treatment or surgery; don't give up hope. Finally, don't go back to bad eating habits and lack of exercise. Heart disease is a wake-up call that you need to change some things in your life. And when you do, you'll be stronger than ever. I use the Capitol steps when I go in to vote now. I climb them instead of using the elevator. It's a small thing, but it's important to me.

After my bypass surgery, I had a bout with depression. I kept thinking how they had busted open my chest, filled me with morphine, split my leg open to take some veins out, and then put them in my heart and sewed it up. The aftermath of that is very emotional. After the surgery, the doctors explained that this sort of reaction is common (they didn't have time to explain this to me before the surgery). They wanted to put me on antidepressants, but I wouldn't do it. I was already taking so many pills and I didn't want any more.

One day, I was on the floor of Congress waiting for a vote and I had tears in my eyes because I was still battling depression. There are House physicians who are assigned to be there and watch the action on the floor in the event someone needs medical assistance. One of them saw the tears in my eyes and walked over and told me to come to his office. After the vote I went there—it was just one level below—and he examined me and kept looking at me, and I just kept on crying. He told me my depression wasn't unusual and it could be eradicated, but I needed to take some antidepressants. I refused, explaining that

I was already taking so many pills now—one to keep my blood from clotting, one to keep my cholesterol down, one for high blood pressure, and on and on. I never did take antidepressants, but the crying jags happen even now. I'll just break down and start crying and I won't even know it's coming.

I'm still trying to eat a better diet. I'm determined to eat more fruits and vegetables, like broccoli and stuff like that. But one of my major challenges is my traveling. It's hard to carry steamed vegetables with me, and if I buy them and leave them in the refrigerator while I'm gone, they're spoiled by the time I get home again. I know how this sounds, and the fact is I'm too lazy to get it together. But I'm working on this because I want to live as long as I can.

Heart disease is the leading cause of death among women, and Black women are at even greater risk. Two things happened to me after my open heart surgery that to this day I can't get over. A girlfriend of mine had been working for the government, and they began to try to get rid of her. I call it "being dogged out by your superiors." Instead of firing you and having to pay severance, they just make your life as miserable as they can so you'll just quit. She wanted an appointment with me to see if I could do anything. And then I looked at the paper one morning before I came back to Indianapolis and there was her obituary. Her husband said she had been feeling bad, so she called her doctor and they set her up for an appointment a week later. It was too late. Another lady had been writing me about how bad she was feeling while working on another federal job and she needed my help. Well, before I could get in touch with her, she died. Both of them had heart disease.

As African American women, we have to begin to define our priorities, and, of course, our health has to come first. We need to pay attention to symptoms; we need to take care of ourselves. We also need to realize that not everyone has the same symptoms; some have tingling in their hands or feet, some have chest pain, some have episodes where they feel like they have gas in their stomachs. Thankfully, the emergency rooms are finally starting to become more sensitive to this.

Still, if a fat man goes into the ER and a Black woman goes into the ER and they have the same symptoms, many times the doctors will immediately check the fat man for heart problems but they'll dismiss the Black woman as having stress. Now doctors are starting to come around and that's good. Today, most are aware that women, and especially Black women, have heart problems, and most doctors are no longer as likely to dismiss their symptoms. Now they check them. That didn't happen to me. I had to tell them that I thought my ticker was gonna blow. Let my story be an example: Don't be afraid to stick up for yourself if you think you're not getting the medical attention you need.

Today, I tend not to sweat the small stuff like I used to do before the surgery. Every minute of the day is a blessing. Every minute is a gift. What I do more of, although I've always done it, is give more. That's money. That's time. That's counsel. That's participation. And I'm just more sensitive now. I've come to understand that you are never going to see a Brink's truck follow a hearse to the cemetery. It's not right to be given a new life and not turn around and try to help somebody else with theirs. I've always been a chump for giving, but I go out of bounds now.

I try to talk people into living instead of giving up because your mind does make things happen one way or another. I think there are a lot of cases where having a positive attitude gives you the extra boost that will help you through an illness.

Lifestyles and habits make a difference with heart disease. It's how you live and how you take care of yourself that makes a difference. So I'm happy to see that more and more people are exercising and paying attention to what they eat. And I'm working at being one of those people.

❧

The Doctor's Notes:
WHEN SURGERY IS URGENT

DANIEL BECKMAN, M.D., cardiac surgeon at Methodist Hospital in Indianapolis

In the emergency room, Julia underwent an angiogram that indicated she had very extensive coronary artery disease. She had severe blockages of several blood vessels. Julia didn't have classic angina before coming into the hospital, but upon arrival she did say her chest was feeling heavy. In addition, the EKG that was performed upon her arrival in the ER suggested that she was already having pre-infarction (pre–heart attack) changes.

This is evidenced by elevations in certain sections of the electrocardiogram that indicate the heart is suffering from a lack of bloodflow. At this point in time, she was in trouble and clearly needed immediate help.

We were giving Julia intravenous medications to treat the angina and to try and quiet down her heart, but they weren't helping, so we decided very quickly that she needed bypass surgery as soon as possible. I told her this wasn't an elective operation. I explained that she had a choice: She could have the bypass surgery and we would get this problem ameliorated, or she could continue to be tired and to have chest pains and all of this would eventually lead to a very large heart attack that might end her career. That's when she looked at me and asked if I was a Republican or a Democrat! I said, "Ms. Carson, it really doesn't matter right now."

I did tell her family she had advanced coronary artery disease. She did very well during the surgery, but about 5 days later she had a mild stroke. Our vascular surgeons evaluated her and realized she had a high-grade blockage in her carotid artery. This is a clot that reduces or cuts off bloodflow to the brain, causing strokes, so we needed to do another procedure to take care of it.

After leaving the hospital, Julia went to Washington, but she felt so ill that she returned to the hospital. She had a second carotid artery that was blocked, so we went in again. She did fine considering the fact she had three major operations in a short period of time. Her prognosis is good, but, as I say to every patient, you have to take care of yourself. She understands this and knows she has to deal with stress and watch her diet. ■

Depression and Recovery

Studies show that about 20 percent of people who have had a major cardiac event such as a heart attack or bypass surgery will experience major depression, usually within a matter of months or weeks after the event. And approximately another 20 percent will experience "transient depression"—a more minor level of behavior change that comes and goes over the first few months after the event.

We don't yet know what causes depression after a cardiac event. Some researchers believe there might be a link to the use of anesthesia during bypass surgery, but more research is needed.

Interestingly, studies reveal that at least 50 percent of patients with heart disease who are depressed were also depressed at least once before they developed heart disease. We don't know how many people with depression go on to develop heart disease, but we do know that depression does increase the risk for developing heart disease and increases the risk of death in those who have heart disease. If you have a heart attack and you are also depressed, you are two to four times more likely to die than someone who has the same disease but isn't depressed.

If you or someone you love has just suffered a heart attack or has undergone heart surgery, be on the lookout for the following common symptoms of depression:

A change in mood. For example, an individual who is normally upbeat will suddenly become sad, quiet, and discordant.

Men, in particular, will become irritable. Usually, the negative mood doesn't last for an extended amount of time; but if it does, this should be considered major depression.

Lack of concentration. Depressed individuals will show a loss of interest in things they used to find exciting. For instance, a baseball fan may not care if a game is on TV.

Sleeplessness. Patients may develop sleeping problems that they didn't have prior to surgery. In many cases, they will wake early and not be able to get back to sleep.

Hopelessness. A depressed person may show no enthusiasm for the future or may not believe that she will ever fully recover. Often, the individual will refuse to take her medication, since she believes that doing so isn't going to help her get better.

Loss of appetite. Someone battling depression may not be hungry at lunch and may only nibble at food during dinner.

The good news is that you don't have to live with depression after a heart attack or heart surgery. Many people find that cardiac rehabilitation classes help them work through their depression. With mild depression, knowing that others are struggling with the same thing can be helpful. In addition, exercise is an excellent antidepressant. Unfortunately, patients with severe depression don't typically attend cardiac rehab classes. Antidepressants should certainly be considered for patients with major depression. Psychotherapy has also been found to be effective, especially if a patient prefers this type of treatment over taking another drug.

—ROBERT CARNEY, M.D., *professor of psychiatry at Washington University School of Medicine in St. Louis, Missouri, who has conducted more than 30 separate studies on the link between heart disease and depression*

Photo Credits

Photographs of the celebrities on the following pages are reprinted with permission, as follows:

Larry King on page xvi, courtesy of Westwood One

Peggy Fleming on page 12, photograph by Harry Langdon

Mike Wallace on page 24, courtesy of CBS News

Kate Jackson on page 34, courtesy of Kate Jackson

Tommy Lasorda on page 50, © 1996 Los Angeles Dodgers, Inc.

Larry King on page 66, courtesy of Westwood One

Pat Buchanan on page 78, courtesy of MSNBC

Eddie Griffin on page 96, courtesy of William Morris Agency

Brian Littrell and family on page 108, courtesy of Brian Littrell

Victoria Gotti on page 128, © Evan Agostini/Staff/Getty Images

Ed Bradley on page 150, courtesy of Tony Esparza for CBS News

Larry King on page 162, photograph by Gregory Heisler. © 2004. Cable News Network. A Time Warner Company. All Rights Reserved.

Phyllis Diller on page 170, photograph by Mark Raboy

Mike Ditka on page 182, courtesy of the Ditka Corporation

Walter Cronkite on page 198, courtesy of CBS/Steve Friedman

Larry King and son on page 208, © Kevin Winter/Getty Images

Louie Anderson on page 220, courtesy of Louie Anderson

Joyce Carol Oates on page 226, photograph by Marion Ettlinger

Mike Medavoy on page 234, photograph by Alia

Regis Philbin on page 244, © Buena Vista Television

Sid Caesar on page 250, courtesy of Sid Caesar

Julia Carson on page 262, courtesy of the House gallery

INDEX

Underscored page references indicate boxed text.

C

Caesar, Sid
angiogenesis in, 253, 260
career of, 251
heart problems of
arrhythmia, 252–53, 257
attitude after, 252, 253,
256–57, 258
bypass surgery for, 253–55
recovery from, 255–57, 259
Caffeine, avoiding, with
tachycardia, 233
Cannom, David, 255
on patient control of health,
257–61
Cardiac arrest, sudden, 147–49
Cardiac rehabilitation classes,
47, 120–21, 122, 167, 195,
196–97, 275
Cardiologists, questions to ask,
206–7
Cardiomyopathy
types of, 143–44
of Victoria Gotti, 130–42, 143,
144
Carney, Robert, on depression
after cardiac event,
274–75
Carotid artery blockage, 267,
268, 273
Carson, Julia
artery blockages of
diagnosis of, 272–73
surgeries for, 266–67, 268,
273
symptoms of, 264, 265–66
attitude change in, 271–72
career of, 263
lifestyle changes of, 270
postsurgical depression of,
269–70

Carson, Tom, 110, 112, 113
on treating Brian Littrell,
123–25
Cell salvage, in heart surgery,
84–85
Checkups, medical, importance
of, 58, 59, 190–91
Cheney, Dick, 213–14
Chest discomfort, as heart attack
symptom, 48, 54, 57, 184,
188, 271. See also Angina;
Pain
Children
heart health and, xii–xiii
with heart problems, advice
for, 118–19
Cholesterol
HDL and LDL, 19
high, as heart disease risk
factor, 14–15, 17–18,
19–20
lowering, 16–18, 21
stress increasing, 23
understanding measurements
of, 19–20
Chronic disease, limitations
from, 214–15, 216
Comedy, recovery and,
176–77
Concentration problems, as
symptom of depression,
275
Congestive heart failure, 22,
174–75
Connolly, Heidi, on dangers of
fen-phen, 242–43
Cooper, John R., Jr., on
breathing tube, 94–95
Cousins, Norman, 258
CPR, 149
C-reactive protein (CRP) tests,
249

Cronkite, Walter
  career of, 199
  heart surgery of, 201–3
    recovery from, 200, 203–4
    symptoms before, 200–201
CRP tests, 249

D

Deaths from heart disease, x
Defibrillator
  automatic external, 147–49
  inspection of, 138–39, 146
  living with, 145–46
  of Victoria Gotti, 137–39, 142
Depression after cardiac event,
    45, 47, 146, 168, 204,
    207, 240, 269–70, 274
  symptoms of, 274–75
  treatment of, 275
Diabetes, as heart disease risk
    factor, 20, 22
Diet
  for cholesterol control,
    16–18
  healthy choices in, 72,
    118–19, 178, 189, 190,
    225, 248, 255, 270
  high-fat
    alternatives to, 190
    as heart disease risk factor,
      21, 100, 102, 104, 247
    questions about, 207
Diller, Phyllis
  career of, 171
  heart problems of, 172–74
    congestive heart failure,
      174–75
    pacemaker for, 174–75,
      181

recovery from, 175–79
  Sick Sinus Syndrome,
    180
  laughter in recovery of,
    176–77, 178
Disease, reactions to, xi
Ditka, Diana, on promoting
    heart health, 188–89
Ditka, Mike
  career of, 183
  heart attacks of, 184–89,
    191–93
    attitude after, 189, 191
    lifestyle changes after, 189,
      190–91
    recovery after, 193–95
    symptoms of, 184–85, 187,
      188–89
Doctors
  advice about, 115, 254
  communication with,
    258
  questions to ask, 27, 39–40,
    206–7
Drysdale, Don, 56

E

EKG, 6, 48, 60, 105,
    272–73
Emotionalism, after heart
    surgery, 91, 168,
    204
Endotracheal tube, in heart
    attack treatment, 105
Ergotamine, heart valve
    damage from, 242
Estrogen
  for cholesterol control, 18
  heart disease risk and, 49

Exercise
  after cardiac event, 190, 225,
    247–48, 255
  in cardiac rehabilitation
    classes, 122, 195,
    196–97
  for depression, 275
  from everyday activity, 91
  questions about, 206–7
  recommended amount of,
    21
  for tachycardia prevention,
    232, 233
  walking as, 72, 89, 157, 255,
    256
External cardiac pacer, in heart
  attack treatment, 106

F

Fallon, Sandra, 174, 175
  on positive attitude,
    176–77
  on Sick Sinus Syndrome,
    180–81
Family history, as heart disease
  risk factor, 14–16,
    17–18, 21, 23, 103, 154,
    156, 223
Fats, dietary. See also High-fat
  diet
  healthy vs. unhealthy, 21
Fear, heart disease and, ix, 195,
    210–12, 241
Fen-phen, heart damage from,
    236–37, 242–43
Fiber
  in healthy diet, 190
  for lowering cholesterol, 21
Fish, omega-3 fatty acids in, 21

Fleming, Peggy
  career of, 13
  diet of, 16–17
  family health history of,
    14–16, 17–18
Fuster, Valentin, 153–54, 155,
    158
  on treating Ed Bradley,
    159–61

G

Garcia, Jorge, 85–86
Gotti, Victoria
  cardiomyopathy of, 130,
    142–43, 144
  defibrillator for, 137–39,
    142
  diagnosis of, 139–40
  pregnancy complications
    with, 131–37
  career of, 129
Griffin, Eddie
  career of, 97
  heart attack of, 98–101
  lifestyle changes after,
    102–4

H

Handler, Martin, 138
  on cardiomyopathy, 142–44
  on defibrillator, 145–46
Happiness, importance of, for
  heart patient, 178
Hayes, Sharonne, on women
  and heart disease,
    40–41

Hazen, Stanley, on
myeloperoxidase test,
248–49
Health insurance, Americans
lacking, 218
Heart attack(s)
emergency treatment of, 7, 9,
105–7, 192
importance of quick treatment
for, 8, 58
personal accounts of
Eddie Griffin, 98–101
Larry King, 2–7, 9–11
Mike Ditka, 184–89
Tommy Lasorda, 52–53
symptoms of, 4–5, 48, 52,
53, 54, 57, 59–60,
98–99, 184–85, 187,
188–89, 271
test for predicting, 248–49
in women, 22, 40–41, 46–47,
48, 271
Heartbeat irregularities
arrhythmia, 138, 145, 237–38,
252–53, 257
pacemaker for, 30–31
in Sick Sinus Syndrome,
173–74, 180–81
tachycardia, 228–33
Heart disease. *See also specific
types*
advances in treatment of,
xi–xii
causes of, xii
deaths from, x
reactions to, xi
risk factors for, 19
anger, 256, 257
diabetes, 20, 22
education about, 104
family history, 14–16,
17–18, 19–20, 21, 23, 103,
154, 156, 223

high blood pressure, 20
high cholesterol, 14–15,
17–18, 19–20
high-fat diet, 21, 100, 102,
104, 247
inactivity, 21
obesity, 21
smoking, 20–21, 22, 104
stress, 23, 100, 103, 156,
186, 256
in women, 22, 40–41, 46–47,
48–49, 270–71
Heart patients
advice for, 115, 118–19, 189,
241, 255, 268–69
in control of health, 257–59
Heart surgery. *See also* Bypass
surgery; Heart valve
surgery
anemia and, 85
avoiding postponement of,
90–91, 91, 114–15
breathing tube after, 87,
94–95, 117, 164, 224
depression after, 45, 47, 146,
168, 204, 207, 240,
269–70, 274–75
future of, xii, 169
preparing for, 90, 115
transfusion with, 84–85
in women, 22
Heart valve damage, from
fen-phen, 236–37,
242–43
Heart valves, replacement,
types of, 87, 93
Heart valve surgery, 92–93
antibiotics after, 93
anticoagulation after, 87, 93
personal accounts of
Brian Littrell, 116–17
Mike Medavoy, 238
Pat Buchanan, 87–92

Heparin, in heart attack
    treatment, 106
High blood pressure
    as heart disease risk factor, 20
    understanding measurement
        of, 20
High cholesterol, as heart
    disease risk factor, 14–15,
    17–18, 19–20
High-fat diet
    alternatives to, 190
    as heart disease risk factor,
        21, 100, 102, 104, 247
Hole in the heart. *See also*
    Ventricular septal defect
    oxygen deprivation from,
        38–39
    symptoms of, 36–37
Holter monitor, 29
Hopelessness, as symptom of
    depression, 275

I

Inactivity, as heart disease risk
    factor, 21
Infection risk, after heart valve
    replacement, 93
Isom, Wayne O., 73, 75–76, 153,
    155, 160, 166, 167, 169,
    199, 201, 203, 212
    on bypass surgery, 204–5
    on heart disease, ix–xiii

J

Jackson, Kate
    career of, 35
    heart problem of, 36–39

heart surgery of, 39–43
    recovery from, 43–46
    on women and heart disease,
        46–47

K

Katz, Richard, 6, 10, 71, 72,
    73
    on heart attack treatment,
        105–7
King, Larry
    childhood of, 217
    on chronic disease, 214–15,
        216
    on fear, 210–12
    heart attack of
        diagnosis of, 5–7
        lifestyle before, 3
        recovery after, 68–72
        symptoms of, 4–5
        treatment of, 7, 9
        warning signs of, 4, 9–10,
            11
    heart surgery of
        angioplasty after, 216
        awareness of health after,
            168–69
        events preceding,
            72–76
        preparation for, 76–77
        recovery from,
            164–68
    on "Hollywood" heart attacks,
        2–3
    Larry King Cardiac
        Foundation of, 218, 219
    on productivity after heart
        surgery, 216–17
Krucoff, Mitchell, on power of
    prayer, 126–27

L

Lanoxin, for tachycardia, 233
Larry King Cardiac Foundation,
    218, 219
Lasorda, Tommy
    career of, 51
    heart attack of, 52–53
        diet after, 57–58
        recovery from, 53–57
Laughter, recovery and, 177, 258
Levy, Warren, 6, 7, 10, 71
Lidocaine, in heart attack
    treatment, 106
Lifestyle changes
    for preventing heart disease,
        71–72, 102–4, 247–48,
        270, 272
    reducing health damage, 190
Lipid profile, 19–20
Littrell, Brian
    Brian Littrell Healthy Heart
        Club for Kids and, 118
    heart surgery of, 113–17,
        124–25
        attitude after, 122–23
        prognosis after, 125
        recovery after, 117, 120–21
        return to stage after,
            121–22
    ventricular septal defect of,
        109–13
Littrell, Jackie, on children with
    heart problems, 118–19

M

Matos, Jeffrey, 27, 29
    on pacemakers, 30–33
McMahon, Don, 56–57

Medavoy, Mike
    career of, 235
    heart problem of
        attitude after, 236, 239, 241
        heart valve surgery for, 238
        pacemaker for, 238–39, 240
        recovery after, 240–41
        symptoms of, 237–38
Medications. *See also specific*
    drugs
    questions about, 206
Melman, Michael, 52–53
Menopause, cardiac risk after, 49
Mitral valve prolapse, 130, 140,
    227
Mood change, as symptom of
    depression, 274–75
Myeloperoxidase (MPO) test, for
    predicting heart attack,
    248–49

N

Nasogastric tube, after heart
    surgery, 95
Nausea, as heart attack
    symptom, 54, 59, 60
Nitroglycerin, in heart disease
    treatment, 48, 99, 106, 153

O

Oates, Joyce Carol
    career of, 227
    tachycardia of, 227, 228–29
        diagnosis of, 231–33
        first attack of, 230–31
        preventing, 232, 233

284   INDEX

Obesity, as heart disease risk
factor, 21
Omega-3 fatty acids, in fish, 21
Orogastric tube, after heart
surgery, 95

P

Pacemakers, 30–33
checking, 28–29, 33, 138–39,
239
defibrillator with, 138–39,
145
implantation of, 27–28, 31
patient restrictions with, 28,
32
personal accounts of
Mike Medavoy, 238–39,
240
Mike Wallace, 26–30, 31
Phyllis Diller, 174–75,
181
Victoria Gotti, 138–39
replacement of, 28, 32–33
risks of, 31
for Sick Sinus Syndrome,
181
Pain, as heart attack symptom,
4–5, 48, 52, 54, 188, 271.
See also Angina; Chest
discomfort
Patient control of health,
257–59
Philbin, Regis
artery blockage of,
246–49
career of, 245
Pohost, Gerald, 37–38, 39
on women and heart disease,
48–49

Prayer, power of, 126–27, 188,
224
Pregnancy, heart disease and,
131–37
Productivity, after heart surgery,
122, 216–17
Psychotherapy, for depression,
275
Pulmonary embolism, 156,
160–61

Q

Questions to ask cardiologist,
27, 39–40, 206–7

R

Reid, Anthony, 53, 57
on treating Tommy Lasorda,
59–62
Restenosis, 65
Rheumatic fever, 130, 140,
143
Risk factors for heart disease,
19
anger, 256, 257
diabetes, 20, 22
education about, 104
family history, 14–16, 17–18,
19–20, 21, 23, 103, 154,
156, 223
high blood pressure, 20
high cholesterol, 14–15,
17–18, 19–20
high-fat diet, 21, 100, 102,
104, 247
inactivity, 21

V

Ventricular fibrillation, 148,
149
Ventricular septal defect,
109–13
Vulnerability, after heart attack,
189, 195

W

Walking, after heart surgery,
72, 89, 157, 255,
256
Wallace, Leighanne, 114–15,
115, 116, 117
Wallace, Mike
career of, 25
pacemaker of, 26–30, 31

Waters, Jonathan, on blood
donations and cell
salvage, 84–85
White, Roger D., on automatic
external defibrillator,
147–49
Women
African-American, heart
attacks in, 22, 270–71
delayed heart attack treatment
in, 8
fen-phen use in, 243
heart attack symptoms in, 48,
271
heart disease in, 22, 40–41,
46–47, 48–49, 270–71

Z

Zeiger, Marty, 212–13